Chair Yoga for Seniors Over 60: Advance Your Wellness

by Riley Miller

Achieve Mobility, Balance, and Weight Loss in just 10 Minutes per Day.

Table of Contents

<u>About Author</u>

After twenty years of practicing yoga, Riley Miller has initiated a chair yoga program with access and wellness for everybody in mind. At the center where she practices, she has nurtured a developing, nourishing atmosphere that integrates traditional yoga principles with a contemporary application for seniors. So, the initiative of chair yoga thus fills a missing part in making yoga accessible and beneficial for people with physical limitations. Therefore, Riley advocates inclusion in the yoga community and offers adapted practices that maintain, and often improve, overall strength, flexibility, and mental clarity for a truly diverse audience.

Her approach to chair yoga transcends only the physical adaption and aspires to fill the hole in accessibility for those searching for holistic benefit. Riley's philosophy undergirds her belief that all should embrace yoga, adapting practices to meet individual needs while holding the essence of the practice toward mind-body-spirit integration. Her work encompasses adapted postures and breathing exercises, meditation[1], and mindfulness. Riley's work heavily contributed to a community where people are uplifted, cared for, and highly regarded—going beyond physical exercises to an integrated wellbeing activity. The book articulates the journey and gives the readers insights into how one can move through aging with grace and vitality through the practice of Chair Yoga. It integrates the core principles of traditional Yoga with their practical applications, delineating a holistic approach that finds resonance with the realities of modern life.

<u>Disclaimer</u>

This book's content aims to complement, not substitute, the patient-healthcare professional relationship and serves strictly educational purposes. Riley Miller, the creator, does not offer medical advice and lacks certification as a healthcare provider. Readers should consult a licensed healthcare provider before beginning any new fitness program, especially if they have injuries, pre-existing medical conditions, or other health concerns.

The poses and wellness techniques described in "Chair Yoga for Seniors" are meant to be a reference for people who want to improve their health by doing mild, chair-based yoga. Although the author has made every effort to guarantee the safety and possible efficacy of the exercises outlined, no guarantee as to the outcome is provided. Results may differ from person to person. Thus, it's essential to modify yoga poses to fit the talents and limits of each practitioner.

Riley Miller disclaims any responsibility for adverse outcomes arising from using the material in this book, whether directly or indirectly. Using this guide, you agree to release Riley Miller from any claims or causes of action, acknowledge that you are engaging in these activities freely, and accept all risks of personal damage.

You should use this book as one tool among many in a balanced lifestyle to achieve health and wellness. We encourage you to listen to your body, move at your own pace, and explore the numerous benefits of mindful movement and breathing on your unique chair yoga journey.

<u>Please do not use this book's information if you disagree with these terms.</u>

I want to highlight to you, our esteemed reader, how crucial personal accountability is to your journey toward physical exercise. Your engagement with the methods and activities in this book demonstrates your dedication to enhancing your overall health and well-being. But it's important to understand that every person's body is different, so what works for one might not work for another. Recognizing and honoring your physical boundaries and requirements is highly recommended.

With a series of mild chair-based yoga practices, this book, "Chair Yoga for Seniors," seeks to improve your physical and emotional well-being. Although we make every effort to offer helpful and secure instructions, you must ensure that each exercise is appropriate for your current level of fitness and health. Remember that this is your journey; make it fit your body, abilities, and objectives. Make the most of chair yoga's reviving and inspiring techniques as you embrace this trip with self-awareness and mindfulness.

Introduction

Every journey begins with a purpose: a spark that fuels our curiosity and drives us onward. In "Chair Yoga for Seniors Over 60," Riley Miller illuminates this spark as the belief that age is merely a number, not a limit to one's abilities or joy.

Within these pages, readers are beckoned not just toward the physical poses of yoga but into a deeper understanding of why movement is essential. It's a quest for harmony in health and personal values, where each posture and breath stands as a testament to a commitment to a well-balanced and vibrant life.

Chair Yoga unveils the mechanisms of movement, offering freedom and strength that defy the years. Guided by Riley Miller's expertise, this book provides the insights necessary for a life enriched by better health and a brighter spirit.

Chapter 1: About Yoga

This chapter delves into the rich history of yoga, tracing back over 5,000 years, to explore its evolution from a profoundly spiritual discipline to a global phenomenon encompassing a broad spectrum of practices. Here, we introduce chair yoga — a specialized form tailored for seniors and individuals with limited mobility. Chair yoga stands out for its accessibility and adaptability, making yoga's benefits available to everyone, regardless of physical condition.

Exploring the Essence of Yoga: Yoga is a pursuit of balanced living that harmonizes the mind, body, and spirit. It advocates for self-awareness, mindfulness, and purposeful living, rooted in ancient wisdom, extending beyond physical exercises, including asanas[2]. All yoga forms, including chair yoga, are grounded in these principles, guiding practitioners toward serenity and insight.

Chair Yoga: Bridging Accessibility and Wellness: Chair Yoga, designed to meet the unique needs of older adults and individuals with mobility challenges, modifies traditional asanas to be performed while seated. This adaptation ensures the practice remains inclusive, enhancing strength, flexibility, and balance. It exemplifies yoga's universal appeal, promising improved physical health, mental clarity, and spiritual connection for practitioners of all ages.

Benefits of Chair Yoga for Seniors: Maintaining an active lifestyle becomes increasingly challenging due to natural body changes as we age. Chair yoga addresses these challenges head-on, offering:

Increased Flexibility and Mobility: Regular practice helps maintain joint fluidity and muscle elasticity, which are crucial for everyday activities.

Enhanced Strength and Balance: Focusing on muscle strengthening and balance reduces the risk of falls, a common concern among seniors.

The Advantages of Senior Chair Yoga

Maintaining physical activity is essential as we age, but it gets more complex because our bodies change. Chair yoga addresses the complexities of maintaining physical activity as we age and respond to changes in our bodies by offering the following benefits:

Increased Flexibility and Mobility: Consistent practice contributes to preserving joint suppleness and muscular elasticity, which are necessary for day-to-day functioning.

Enhanced Strength and Balance: Seniors often worry about falling, but chair yoga helps strengthen muscles and improve balance.

Stress Reduction and Mental Clarity: Like other styles of yoga, chair yoga includes breathing techniques and meditation to help lower stress and enhance focus and mental clarity. Yoga and meditation can help people deal with and relieve short-term and long-term stress. They can also help people with diseases deal with other problems that come with them and improve their quality of life[1].

Pain Relief: It can also help with the pain and suffering from age-related illnesses such as osteoporosis, arthritis, and other ailments. Many studies have demonstrated that asana, meditation, or both can improve flexibility and functional mobility[3] in individuals suffering from a variety of chronic pain[4] conditions while also reducing pain and disability. In some cases, practitioners have even managed to reduce or altogether discontinue the use of painkillers.

A Comprehensive Strategy for Wellbeing: This practice holistically nurtures mental, emotional, and physical well-being, offering more than just physical exercise. For seniors who may frequently feel alone, the practice promotes mindfulness and provides a sense of community, both of which are essential.

Misconceptions of Chair Yoga

Chair yoga is sometimes thought of as a type solely for older people or people with physical disabilities, although it has far broader applications. This section seeks to dispel these misconceptions and show how open and adaptable chair yoga is. Chair yoga is a comprehensive approach to wellbeing accessible to people of all ages and fitness levels despite the misconception that it is constrained or simplistic. It combines fundamental yoga principles and has both mental and physical health advantages. We will examine how chair yoga presents obstacles and accommodates a range of demands, offering a comprehensive experience that enhances the practice for all participants.

Only the Elderly and Those with Physical Limitations Should Practice Chair Yoga

The idea that chair yoga is only for older people or people with physical impairments is a prevalent fallacy. Although chair yoga is an excellent choice for these populations, its advantages are much more widespread. Chair yoga is accessible to people of all ages and fitness levels. We especially recommend chair yoga to individuals who spend much time sitting at work or who wish to approach yoga more gently. In contrast, chair yoga suits older adults and those with physical limitations well. Its benefits extend to people of all ages and fitness levels.

The "Real" Yoga Practice Isn't Chair Yoga

A common misconception is that chair yoga is less authentic than traditional yoga. This misunderstanding results from the idea that practicing yoga requires difficult, physically taxing postures. Chair yoga is as genuine as any other yoga practice because it incorporates all essential yoga tenets, such as the mind-body connection, breath control, and physical and emotional tranquility development.

Chair Yoga Isn't Hard Enough and Is Too Easy

Some people can underestimate the difficulty of chair yoga because they think it's too simple or mild to be helpful. Chair yoga can be challenging. Practitioners can modify the exercise in chair yoga to increase flexibility, balance, and strength. Far from diminishing the intensity of one's yoga practice, the objective is for practitioners to use the chair to explore and enhance their practice.

There Are No Real Physical Benefits from Chair Yoga

Contrary to common belief, chair yoga has several physical benefits. These advantages are critical for preserving functional independence and general health in elderly and immobile people.

The Only Thing Physical Movement Is in a Chair Yoga

While often perceived as focused on physical postures, chair yoga is inherently holistic, nurturing the mind, body, and spirit equally. The chair yoga practice includes components of meditation and pranayama[5], which are vital for mental and emotional health. It's a practice that takes equal care of the body, mind, and spirit.

It Is Not Possible to Adjust Chair Yoga for Various Skill Levels

Contrary to some beliefs, chair yoga is not a one-size-fits-all practice with limited adaptability. Instructors can adapt chair yoga significantly, making it suitable for beginners and experienced yogis. They can modify poses to match different ability levels and recommend adjustments to simplify or intensify the practice.

Chair Yoga Is Uninteresting or Unrewarding

Finally, there needs to be a better perception that chair yoga is less exciting and monotonous than other types of Yoga. There is no way that this is not the case. Chair yoga sessions may be lively and varied, using a variety of poses and methods to keep the practice fresh and captivating. It provides a unique kind of Yoga that is both challenging and enjoyable.

Transformational Stories for Seniors of Chair Yoga

Yoga is a path of self-discovery and development, not just a physical exercise. Senior citizens practicing chair yoga embody the journey of self-discovery and growth that extends beyond mere physical activity. Their shared stories illustrate this practice's profound impact on their overall wellbeing, mobility, and health, highlighting the numerous advantages[2] of each stretch, breath, and moment of stillness in senior chair yoga.

Margaret's Return to Gardening

At 78 years old, Margaret's arthritis made gardening an excruciating chore. To control her pain, she began chair yoga. She saw a noticeable joint strength and flexibility improvement after a few months. She's back in her garden now, lovingly caring for her roses with less suffering and more happiness, thankful for her rekindled enthusiasm.

Emma's Victory Against Depression

Emma, 72, has suffered from sadness ever since her husband's death. She began going to chair yoga classes after receiving encouragement from her daughter. Her mood steadily improved due to breathing techniques and mild activity. Her daily life seemed joyful once more, and yoga became a source of strength and serenity.

David's Stroke Recuperation

David, 70, had a stroke and experienced severe mobility problems. As part of his rehabilitation, he started chair yoga, determined to reclaim his independence. He eventually regained most of his lost mobility and balance, and he credits chair yoga's focus and soft motions for his recovery.

Leo's Triumph Over Prolonged Back Pain

Leo has suffered from chronic back pain for many years. When he was seventy-four, he found chair yoga and began doing it daily. He could play with his grandchildren and resume hobbies he had given up as his back discomfort gradually decreased.

Helen's Return to Self-Assurance

Helen, eighty years old, felt her confidence waning. Through chair yoga, she learned to embrace her body's potential at any age and found a connection with a supportive community. Her newfound confidence reignited her adventurous spirit and spilled over into other areas of her life.

George's Diabetes Care

George, 67, found it difficult to control his diabetes. Adding chair yoga to his practice and making nutritional adjustments helped tremendously. His doctor saw improvements in his general health and a more steady blood sugar level. George attributes his ability to manage his health to chair yoga.

John's Struggle with Isolation

John, 65, felt alone and disengaged after retiring. He went to a chair yoga class nearby, recommended by a buddy. Yoga improved his physical health, but the class fostered a sense of community and helped him gain new friends. John's circle of acquaintances grew more prominent and more like-minded, and his loneliness diminished.

These personal stories reflect the varied experiences of individuals who have used chair yoga to lead more contented lives. They highlight how chair yoga fosters a strong sense of community and belonging, overcomes physical obstacles, and provides mental and emotional renewal.

Each narrative celebrates the human spirit's adaptability and perseverance, from conquering physical obstacles to embracing a fulfilled existence. Come along as we examine these moving tales highlighting chair yoga's positive effects on older adults' lives.

As we close Chapter 1's discussion of chair yoga and understand its profound effects on mental, spiritual, and physical health, we also acknowledge that holistic health[6] encompasses more than physical activity. Chapter 2 focuses on the essential components of nutrition and hydration, which nourish our bodies and improve our yoga practice. Like chair yoga modifies conventional yoga poses to improve strength and flexibility, eating and drinking mindfully feed and primes our bodies to reap the full advantages of these practices. In Chapter 2, we explore how a customized diet and sufficient water can enhance the benefits of chair yoga, creating a holistic approach to well-being as we age.

Chapter 2: Hydration and Nutrition

As we embrace our golden years and engage in activities like chair yoga, we must tailor our eating habits to our bodies' evolving requirements. This section offers straightforward nutritional advice to bolster your health and energy, ensuring a vibrant and active lifestyle.

Elevating Wellness with Nutritious Eating: Adapting your diet is crucial as you partake in chair yoga and other activities, aligning with your body's shifting needs. Emphasizing nutrient-dense foods ensures that every calorie consumed contributes to your health, compensating for the metabolic rate decline associated with aging.

Maximizing Nutrient Intake: Opt for a nutrient-rich diet that maximizes vitamins, minerals, fiber, and antioxidants per calorie. Whole foods form the cornerstone of such a diet, providing unprocessed, fresh, and wholesome nutrition that includes fruits, vegetables, lean proteins, whole grains, and healthy fats.

Calorie Consumption with Mindfulness: Smart meal choices that pack more nutrients into fewer calories, alongside mindful portion control, can enhance well-being and help maintain a healthy weight. Incorporate lean proteins, whole grains, and a variety of fruits and vegetables to fuel your body optimally for yoga and daily life.

Mindful Eating and Portion Awareness: Practicing portion control by heeding hunger cues and avoiding overeating is a balanced approach to nutrition. This mindful eating helps ensure your body receives the necessary nutrients without excess.

Prioritizing Protein: For seniors, especially those practicing chair yoga, prioritizing protein intake is essential to support muscle health and overall metabolic function. A diverse diet, including Greek yogurt, lean meats, and plant-based options like tofu, ensures a robust protein intake for sustaining muscle strength and vitality.

Essential Nutrients for Aging Bodies: Incorporate calcium-rich foods for bone health and vitamin D from sunlight and fortified sources to support calcium absorption. B vitamins in greens, meats, and grains are crucial for energy, while Omega-3 fatty acids from sources like walnuts and salmon support cognitive and cardiovascular health.

Hydration: A Pillar of Health Hydration is fundamental for health, particularly in seniors engaging in chair yoga. Regular water intake combats dehydration signs like fatigue, ensuring your body functions optimally.

Incorporating water-rich foods into your diet provides hydration and essential nutrients. Aim for at least seven glasses of water daily, adjusting based on individual needs and conditions. Hydration before and after yoga enhances focus and aids recovery, making it a crucial aspect of your wellness routine.

Establish a hydration habit by drinking water daily, using urine color as a hydration indicator. Ensuring adequate water intake is vital for maintaining health, enhancing chair yoga practice, and supporting overall well-being as we age.

Strategic Weight Loss for Chair Yoga Practitioners

Seniors who practice chair yoga must tackle weight loss from a planned and well-rounded standpoint. Understanding that weight loss varies over our senior years due to body composition and metabolic rate modifications is critical. These are the leading suggestions for approaching weight loss securely and efficiently:

Being aware of Metabolic Changes in Seniors:

Recognize Slower Metabolism: Seniors should acknowledge that their metabolism naturally decreases as they age. Although this slowdown means weight loss may happen more gradually than in younger years, consistent effort can still lead to successful outcomes.

Creating Reasonable Weight Loss Objectives:

Adopt a Methodical and Gradual Approach: Aim for steady and gradual weight loss. Rapid weight loss can harm older adults, as it may lead to muscle loss.

Personalized Objectives: Determine attainable objectives based on your lifestyle, mobility, and present state of health. Focusing on your health journey is more important than competing with others.

A Well-Balanced Diet to Lose Weight:

Portion Control: Even while eating healthful meals, be mindful of portion proportions to prevent overindulging.

Nutrient-Dense Foods:

Pay attention to nutrient-dense foods like leafy greens, lean meats, and whole grains that are low in calories.

Reducing Empty Calorie Intake: Cut back on items high in empty calories, such as processed meals, sugary snacks, and too many carbohydrates.

Including Chair Yoga in Programs for Losing Weight:

Frequent Practice: By enhancing metabolism, building muscular tone, and lowering stress—which can occasionally trigger overeating—regular chair yoga practice can help people lose weight.

Mindful Eating and Being Aware of Sugar to Help You Lose Weight

A crucial weight-controlling tactic is mindful eating, which is especially important for senior citizens doing chair yoga. It entails being conscious of hunger cues and eating in reaction to them rather than out of emotions or boredom. This strategy helps avoid overeating and promotes a better relationship with food.

Maintaining hydration is another essential aspect of mindful eating. People often mistake thirst for hunger, leading to unnecessary snacking. Individuals can better manage weight and distinguish between hunger and thirst signals by ensuring regular water intake.

It's also critical to comprehend how sugar affects general health and weight loss. Consuming too much sugar might make it difficult to lose weight because it has little nutritional benefit and can cause energy spikes and crashes. These variations impact chair yoga performance and consistency. Furthermore, consuming too much sugar is linked to a higher risk of developing heart disease and type 2 diabetes. Switching to natural sugar sources, such as fruits, and reducing processed foods with added sugars will help you lose weight and make chair yoga exercises more successful.

In conclusion, weight loss for seniors ought to be a conscious, health-conscious endeavor, particularly for those who practice chair yoga. Making permanent lifestyle modifications that improve general well-being rather than making drastic changes quickly is essential. Remember that everybody is unique and that feeling good about yourself, energized, and at ease in your fantastic body counts most.

The table below provides a standard guideline for optimal body weight based on height for seniors over 60. Remember, these approximations can vary based on gender, body composition, and overall health. It is always best to consult with a healthcare professional for personalized advice.

This is a simplified table:

HEIGHT	IDEAL WEIGHT RANGE (LBS)
5'0"	97 - 127
5'1"	101 - 132
5'2"	106 - 136
5'3"	110 - 141
5'4"	114 - 145
5'5"	118 - 150
5'6"	122 - 155
5'7"	126 - 160
5'8"	130 - 164
5'9"	134 - 169
5'10"	138 - 174
5'11"	142 - 179
6'0"	146 - 184

The unit of measurement for height is feet and inches, or ft and in. For instance, 5'4" denotes 5 feet and 4 inches.

The unit of measurement for weight is pounds or lbs.

These weight ranges have been established based on a healthy body mass index (BMI) for older persons. Adults can be categorized as underweight, overweight, or obese using the BMI, a straightforward weight-for-height index. However, since BMI cannot distinguish between weight gained from muscle and weight gained from fat, it may not be a reliable indicator of body fat in those with high muscle mass.

Recall that your optimum weight is more than simply a number on a scale; it's also a function of your overall health, level of mobility, and energy. A balanced diet and regular exercise, such as chair yoga, are essential for preserving a healthy weight and general well-being.

Guidelines for proper hydration, meals before and after yoga

For the best results, you should wait at least two hours after a full meal before doing chair yoga. This time, it lets your body digest properly, making your yoga exercise more comfortable and practical.

Pre-Yoga Meals: For a rapid energy boost, have a small yogurt or banana around or a small apple with a tablespoon of peanut butter, which provides a good mix of natural sugars and protein, or whole-grain crackers with hummus is a balance of carbohydrates and protein. An excellent choice is a slice of whole-grain bread and avocado for healthy fats and fiber.

Time: 30 to 50 minutes

before your chair yoga class

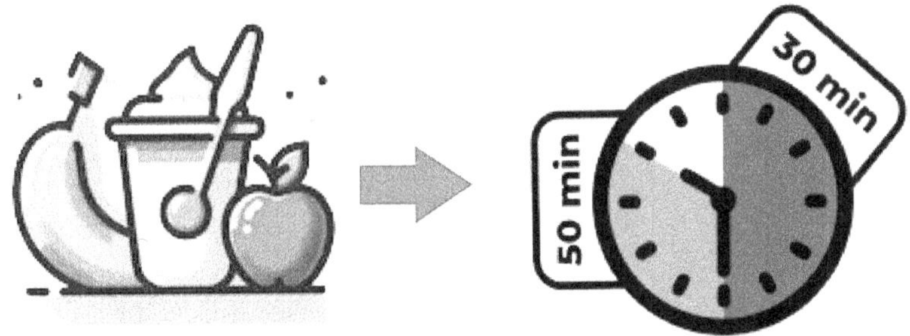

Post-Yoga Meals: To support muscle repair and restore energy reserves, refuel with a balanced meal that includes protein, carbs, and healthy fats after yoga or a turkey and cheese sandwich on whole-grain bread, with a side of carrot sticks, offers a balanced mix of protein, carbs, and veggies.

For a nutrient-rich meal, a salad with grilled chicken, mixed greens, tomatoes, cucumbers, and a vinaigrette dressing.

For a protein-rich meal, scrambled eggs with spinach, mushrooms, and a slice of whole-grain toast.

Avoiding high-sugar snacks or foods is essential, as they can lead to energy crashes and don't provide the sustained energy needed for Yoga. Healthy, balanced meals are vital for maintaining energy levels and supporting the body's needs for yoga practice.

Hydration Guidelines:

Before starting your chair yoga session, it's crucial to consider your hydration. Drinking a glass of water an hour before practice ensures you are well-hydrated, enhancing your physical performance and concentration. Hydration is vital to a successful yoga practice as it helps maintain energy levels and prevents muscle cramps.

After completing your yoga session, it's equally important to rehydrate. Replenish fluids lost during the activity by drinking water or another hydrating, non-caffeinated beverage. This post-exercise hydration aids in recovery and helps maintain your overall health. Remember, staying hydrated is essential to any fitness routine, including chair yoga.

As we've seen, proper nutrition and hydration in your body are crucial for a successful chair yoga practice. But mentally and physically, preparing yourself is just as vital. We move from discussing yoga's physical aspects to going through the power of breathing in Chapter 3. In addition to being an essential component of yoga, breathing, or "pranayama," is a vital tool for improving your general health[3]. The breathing exercises in this next chapter are tailored especially for chair yoga practitioners. They will show you how breathing exercises can significantly impact your physical and mental well-being."

Chapter 3: Breathing Exercises

"Chapter 3 introduces pranayama—essential breathing techniques integral to chair yoga, enhancing physical and emotional health. Pranayama includes guided breath awareness, diaphragmatic breathing, and alternate nostril breathing, each offering unique benefits such as improved lung function, stress reduction, and enhanced focus[3]. We provide easy-to-follow instructions, making these practices accessible to everyone, regardless of yoga experience. By integrating these techniques into daily life, individuals can experience profound improvements in overall well-being. This section guides you in incorporating pranayama into your chair yoga routine, showing how these practices enhance the physical components of yoga for a holistic health approach. You can maximize benefits by pairing them with the mindfulness practices detailed later in this book, thus ensuring a comprehensive enhancement of life quality through chair yoga.

Breathing Techniques for Anytime Use

Breathing exercises from chair yoga can be seamlessly integrated into your daily routine, offering a flexible way to enhance mental clarity, reduce stress, and boost overall health—no need for a physical workout. Chapter 5 of the 28-Day Chair Yoga Challenge dives into detailed instructions for incorporating these techniques, aiming to enrich your practice by blending specific pranayama exercises with yoga poses.

Making these breathing exercises a regular part of your life, whether as independent activities or elements of your chair yoga sessions, promises substantial health benefits. They are vital in improving wellness, reducing stress, and bolstering respiratory health. Embrace pranayama's transformative power to elevate your chair yoga experience, bringing increased vitality and serenity to your journey.

Upon completing Chapter 3, we now deeply understand the role of pranayama in enriching chair yoga. We have explored its numerous health benefits, which include enhancing lung function, reducing stress, and promoting tranquility. Transitioning from theoretical knowledge to practical application, Chapter 4, 'Preparing for Chair Yoga,' guides us in setting up the ideal environment for our practice. This preparation involves selecting the right chair, arranging a supportive space, wearing comfortable clothes, and combining external setup with internal readiness through mindfulness and breathing techniques, all contributing to a comprehensive chair yoga experience.

<u>Chapter 4: Preparing for Chair Yoga</u>

This chapter focuses on preparing for a safe and effective chair yoga experience. It emphasizes the importance of safety precautions, such as creating a clutter-free area and being mindful of physical limitations. Setting up the proper environment is crucial, including choosing a quiet, well-lit, ventilated space. Selecting the right chair is essential for stability and comfort, and wearing appropriate attire ensures ease of movement. This preparation is vital to a fulfilling chair yoga practice, ensuring safety and comfort and maximizing the benefits of your sessions.

Essential guidelines for practicing safety:

Creating a Safe Practice Space: Ensure your yoga space has minimal clutter and sufficient movement room. Reducing clutter and ensuring ample space decreases the risk of accidents and enhances focus during your practice.

Recognizing Your Boundaries: Pay attention to what your body can and cannot do. Always put your safety and comfort first; adjust your positions as necessary, and never force yourself into pain.

Pacing and Rest Periods: Start lightly and build up to moderate intensity over time. Pay attention to your body's cues and rest to avoid exerting too much.

Nutritional and Hydration Considerations: To enhance your yoga practice, apply the dietary guidance in Chapter 2. Energy and concentration mainly depend on eating a healthy diet and staying hydrated.

Mindful Movement and Breathing: To guarantee a steady and balanced practice, enter into each yoga posture with mindfulness and intention. Use your breath as a guide.

Ready for an Emergency: Keep your phone nearby during practice in an emergency. Tell someone about your yoga plan for extra safety, especially if you live alone.

Following these detailed instructions, you can enjoy a secure, comfortable, and effective chair yoga session that boosts your mental and physical health.

Safety is paramount in any physical activity, including chair yoga. Adhering to these precautions ensures a safe and beneficial chair yoga experience, aiming to enhance your physical health, safety, and wellbeing. Chair yoga offers many advantages for seniors; however, it's crucial to approach the practice with care. This chapter outlines necessary safety measures and guidelines to foster a secure environment for chair yoga sessions, allowing you to minimize risks while maximizing the enjoyment and effectiveness of your practice.

Choosing the Right Chair

Choosing the right chair is essential for a secure and productive yoga practice. Take into consideration these important points:

Stability: Choose a chair without wheels to maintain stability during yoga poses.

Height and Support: For good posture, your knees should be at a straight angle, and your feet should be flat on the ground when using the chair. For easy movement and postural support, a firm seat is preferable.

Backrest: To avoid back discomfort, use a backrest that maintains your spine's natural curve.

Armrests: For maximum mobility, chairs without armrests are the best option. Choose a chair with armrests that don't impede movement if balance is an issue.

Material and Maintenance: Preferably, use a material that is easy to clean and long-lasting. Check the chair's safety regularly, mainly if used frequently.

Therefore, your chair is a piece of furniture and a tool that helps you do yoga. Taking the effort to choose the appropriate chair will significantly improve your chair yoga experience. Remember that the most incredible chair for you is stable, comfortable, and meets your specific needs, letting you focus on your practice confidently and efficiently.

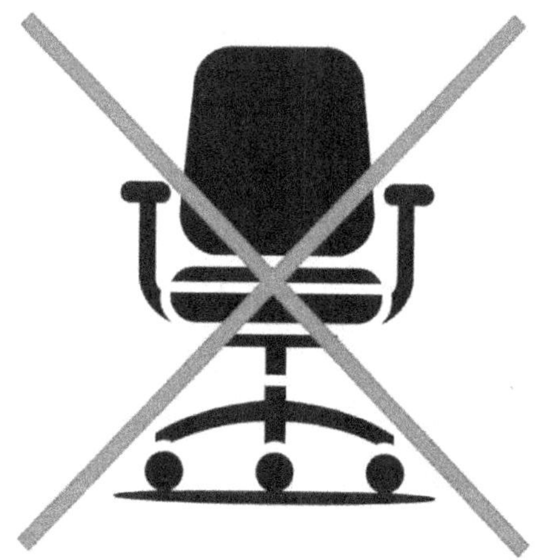

Choose the Right Clothes

The clothing you wear during your chair yoga practice significantly impacts how comfortable and successful your session is. This subchapter explains choosing the correct clothing that blends comfort, utility, and ease of movement to ensure the best yoga experience possible. Remember the following:

Comfort and Mobility: Choose clothing that is both cozy and facilitates simple mobility. The best materials for preserving comfort and flexibility during yoga poses are soft and breathable.

Fit and functionality: Clothes should be loose enough for comfortable movement. Remember that clothing that is too loose could hinder your practice.

Footwear: To keep stability and grip, wear non-slip socks if you'd rather not walk barefoot.

Medical devices and accessories: Minimize jewelry and other accessories to prevent distractions and to guarantee safety. Also, ensure your clothing easily fits any medical equipment you need.

Proper clothing guarantees comfort, safety, and movement flexibility, improving your yoga practice.

In conclusion, selecting appropriate clothing for chair yoga requires balancing comfort, functionality, and personal style. Your gear should facilitate your movements, allow you to Concentrate on your practice, and contribute to a great yoga experience. Remember, the finest yoga clothes make you feel comfortable and will enable you to move and breathe freely.

Bridging Preparation and Practice

Now that you have created an environment outside that is favorable, let's focus inside. Changing from the physical setting to chair yoga is a step toward a holistic health journey that integrates mental and physical well-being. It's not just about switching up your activities; it's also about getting ready for a practice that supports your physical and emotional health. It's time to explore the inner workings of your practice in a safe and comfortable space, emphasizing breathing techniques and mindfulness. This method will give your chair yoga practice a comprehensive beginning.

It's essential to understand how the things we discussed in Chapter 4, "Preparing for Chair Yoga," help you make a suitable space for your practice to fit in with the actual practice of chair yoga. Preparation isn't just about making sure there is enough space; it's also about getting in the right frame of mind and attitude, which are very important for the exercises that are coming up. As we move on to Chapter 5, "Getting Started with Chair Yoga," let's keep the levels of awareness and purpose we've set. We will build our chair yoga practice on this mental and physical readiness to ensure every movement and breath is as valuable and meaningful as possible.

As we wrap up Chapter 4, " Preparing for Chair Yoga," we see how important it is to create an appropriate environment for chair yoga that extends beyond the physical space. Adopting the proper attitude and frame of mind is necessary for the following exercises. As we transition to Chapter 5, "Getting Started with Chair Yoga," we continue to develop the consciousness and intention we have begun. This readiness forms the foundation of our chair yoga practice, making every pose and breath as meaningful as possible.

Chapter 5: Getting Started with Chair Yoga

Chapter 5 continues the exploration of chair yoga's essence, emphasizing mental and physical preparation and building upon the foundational work from Chapter 4, which focuses on creating a conducive physical environment. This chapter stresses the importance of mindfulness and breathing techniques in chair yoga. Establishing a positive practice space sets the stage for enhancing flexibility, strength, and mental well-being. With the external environment prepared, it becomes crucial to turn your attention inward, delving into the core aspects of your chair yoga practice.

Mindfulness and breathing exercises are pivotal to a comprehensive chair yoga routine. They bridge the gap between physical preparation and mental readiness, enriching your practice by fostering a deeper connection to your body and a heightened awareness of each movement. Intentional practice and pranayama (breathing exercises) rejuvenate the body, regulate emotions, and calm the mind, creating a harmonious balance between your mental and physical states. These foundational practices enhance your chair yoga experience and prepare you for the advanced exercises, setting the stage for a transformative journey through chair yoga.

As we progress, incorporating these mindfulness and breathing techniques into your daily routine—especially during the 28-day challenge—is essential. They are not mere additions but integral components that amplify the benefits of your chair yoga practice. Follow the warm-up recommendations and engage with these practices to ensure a comprehensive and rewarding yoga experience.

Mindfulness, Meditation, and Breathing Exercises

Integrating mindful practices, meditation, and controlled breathing into your chair yoga routine enriches your physical and mental well-being. These elements are foundational to the 28-day challenge, transforming it from a simple exercise program into a comprehensive wellness journey. See Chapter 6, "Creating Daily Rituals for a 28-Day Chair Yoga

Challenge," for more detailed practice techniques. Engage in the following methods to deepen your yoga practice:

1. **Creating a Mindful Foundation:**
   - **Start in a Seated Position:** Sit comfortably in your chair, feet flat on the floor, and hands gently resting on your lap.
   - **Embrace the Present Moment Awareness:** Close your eyes and focus on the present moment. Pay attention to any feelings in your body, the rhythm of your breathing, and the sounds around you.
2. **Breathing Exercises to Relax and Focus:**
   - **Diaphragmatic Breathing:** Concentrate on deep abdominal breathing. Inhale slowly, allowing your belly to expand, then exhale gently, feeling the belly sink. This deep breathing method helps both relaxation and mental clarity.
   - **Counted Breath:** Slowly inhale for four counts, hold for two counts, and then exhale for four. This practice helps you control your breathing and concentrate your thoughts.
3. **Integrating conscious Movement: Move with Awareness**: Keep a conscious connection with your body as you move into chair yoga postures. Move carefully and attentively, coordinating each action with your breath.
4. **Visualization and Guided Imagery Meditation:** Peaceful Imagery: Imagine a relaxing sitting setting. Engage your senses in this vision, noticing the sights, sounds, and fragrances of this tranquil setting. This technique promotes a profound sense of peace.
5. **Incorporating Meditation After Practice:** Seated Meditation: Return to a seated position after finishing your yoga poses. To end your exercise peacefully, engage in a brief meditation focusing on your breath or maintaining your imagery.
6. **Developing a Regular Practice:** Daily Mindfulness and Breathing Exercises: Set aside a few minutes daily for these practices. Consistent engagement improves mental clarity, reduces stress, and supplements your physical yoga practice.

Incorporating mindfulness, meditation, and breathing techniques into your chair yoga program promotes overall wellness. These activities improve the physical benefits of yoga and promote mental and emotional well-being, resulting in a harmonic balance in your daily life.

Adopting these practices ensures a holistic approach to chair yoga, blending physical exercises with mental and emotional wellness strategies. As you progress through the 28-Day Chair Yoga Challenge, seamlessly incorporate these techniques to achieve a balanced and enriched yoga experience.

Poses of chair yoga

We designed this section to introduce readers to the adapted poses that form the core of chair yoga classes, ensuring they are accessible and easy for practitioners of all levels. While subsequent sections will detail the 28-Day Challenge with comprehensive instructions for each pose, our goal here is to familiarize you with the essence and versatility of chair yoga. This approach allows for a seamless integration of yoga into daily life, highlighting yoga's adaptability to meet individuals' diverse needs. Through this exploration, we cultivate a deeper understanding and appreciation for the transformative power of yoga, tailored to the comfort and support of a chair.

Seated Mountain Pose (Tadasana)

The Seated Mountain Pose is vital for enhancing your posture and ensuring your spine is aligned correctly. It forms a foundation for numerous seated yoga movements, emphasizing the creation of a robust and stable base and concentration. In this posture, your head, neck, and spine should align in a straight line, facilitating a better posture and serving as a preparatory stance for other chair-based poses. This tranquil pose fosters breath awareness, is conducive to meditation, and promotes a sense of mental stability and grounding. Aim for stability in the lower body during the pose, with the upper body remaining light and effortless. Imagine your torso and head gently lifting off your lower extremities to achieve this balance. If reaching the floor is difficult, using a prop like books under your feet can help maintain proper alignment, ensuring your thighs stay parallel to the ground and your knees align with your hips. This careful attention to posture and breath prepares you for further exercises and helps you achieve a serene, meditative state.

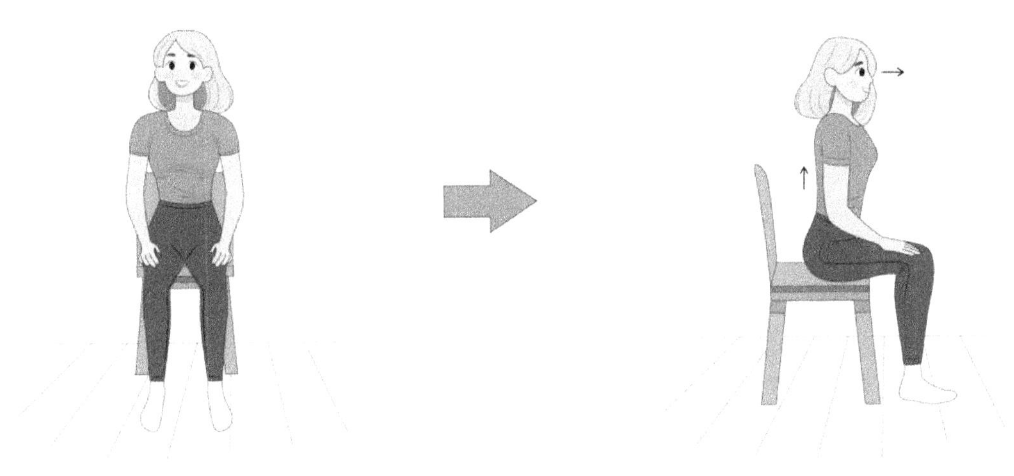

Seated Cat-Cow:

The Seated Cat-Cow stretch is a gentle, accessible exercise that improves flexibility and mobility in the spine while seated. This movement involves alternating between arching the back and rounding the spine, mimicking the movements of a cat stretching and a cow with its head raised. It's excellent for releasing back, neck, and shoulder tension, promoting circulation and spinal health. As you move, inhaling during the cow pose (arched back) and exhaling during the cat pose (rounded spine) helps deepen your focus on breath, enhancing relaxation and mindfulness. This exercise is an easy and self-contained yoga practice for improving posture and body awareness. Regularly incorporating the Seated Cat-Cow stretches into your routine can increase spinal flexibility, improve posture, and reduce back pain, making it a beneficial practice for individuals of all ages and fitness levels.

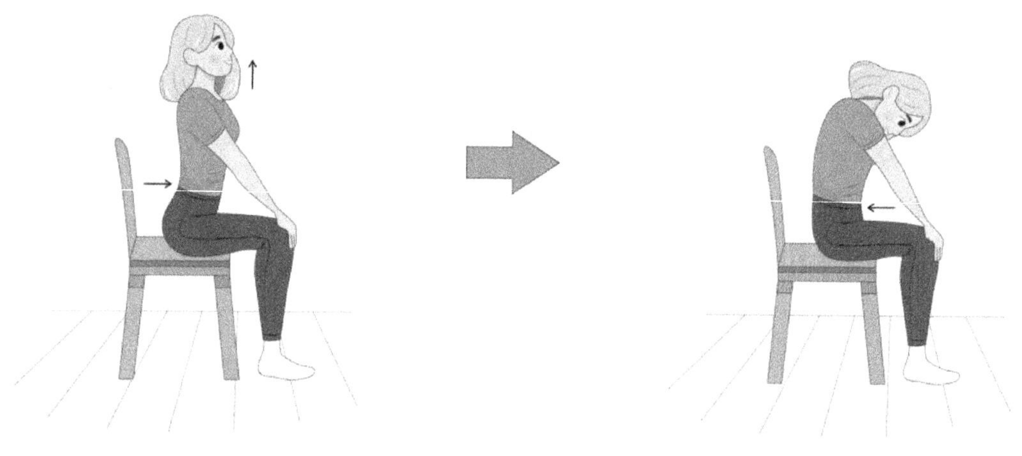

Chair Pigeon Pose:

The Chair Pigeon Pose is a seated yoga position designed to open the hips and increase flexibility. It's an accessible exercise that can be performed in any setting, making it perfect for those with a sedentary lifestyle or anyone looking to ease hip tension. By placing one ankle on the opposite knee while seated, this pose gently encourages the hip joint to open, enhancing mobility and reducing discomfort. It is an essential foundation for hip health, promoting circulation and encouraging a mindful connection to the body's needs and limitations. Additionally, this pose aids in stabilizing the core and maintaining a balanced posture, which can alleviate back pain and improve overall body alignment. Regularly practicing the Chair Pigeon Pose can significantly improve flexibility, posture, and mind-body awareness, making it a staple in seated yoga. This exercise prepares the body for more advanced yoga poses and offers immediate relief from the stress and strain of daily activities.

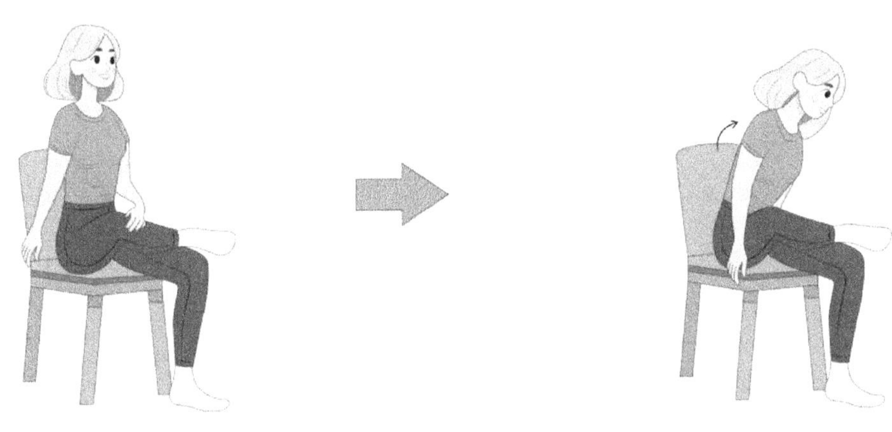

Chair Plank

The Chair Plank Pose, adapted for a seated position, integrates core strengthening and balance into your yoga practice. This variation brings the plank's benefits into an accessible form, focusing on engaging the core, arms, and shoulders without falling on the floor. It's an excellent exercise for building stability and strength in the upper body and core muscles, enhancing posture, and supporting spinal health. By utilizing a chair, this pose allows individuals of all fitness levels to safely practice and gain the posture-improving and muscle-toning advantages of the traditional plank pose. Regular practice of the Chair Plank Pose can contribute to a stronger core, improved balance, and a greater sense of body awareness, making it a valuable addition to any seated yoga routine or exercise regimen.

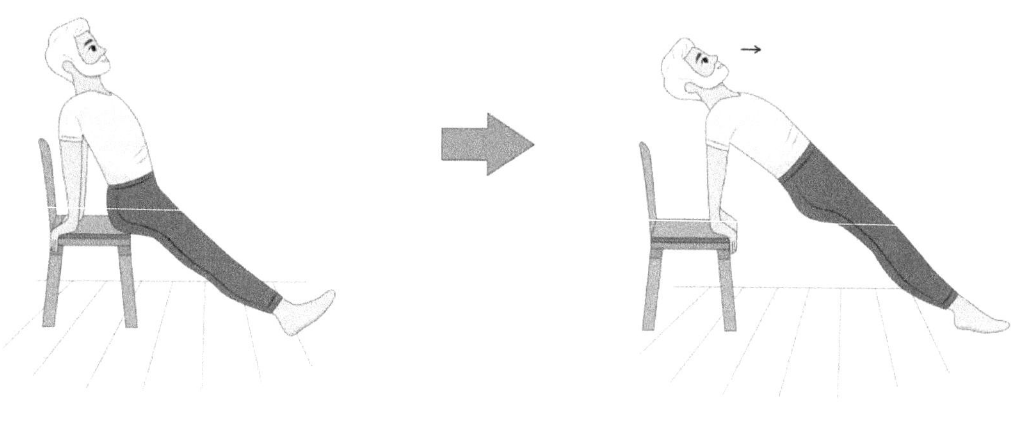

Chair Warrior Poses (I & II)

The Chair Warrior Poses, including Warrior I and Warrior II, adapt the traditional standing versions for seated practice, catering to various abilities with strength, flexibility, and focus. Designers of these poses aim to engage the core, legs, and arms while enhancing posture and concentration. Warrior I focuses on building strength through the torso and shoulders, promoting an upward stretch and engagement of the front body. Warrior II emphasizes lateral flexibility and arm strength, promoting an expansive chest and shoulder alignment. Both poses enhance mental focus and body awareness, making them essential for a comprehensive seated yoga routine. Regular practice can increase muscle tone, improve balance, and create a deeper connection between mind and body, accommodating those who may require or prefer seated exercises.

Chair Warrior I:

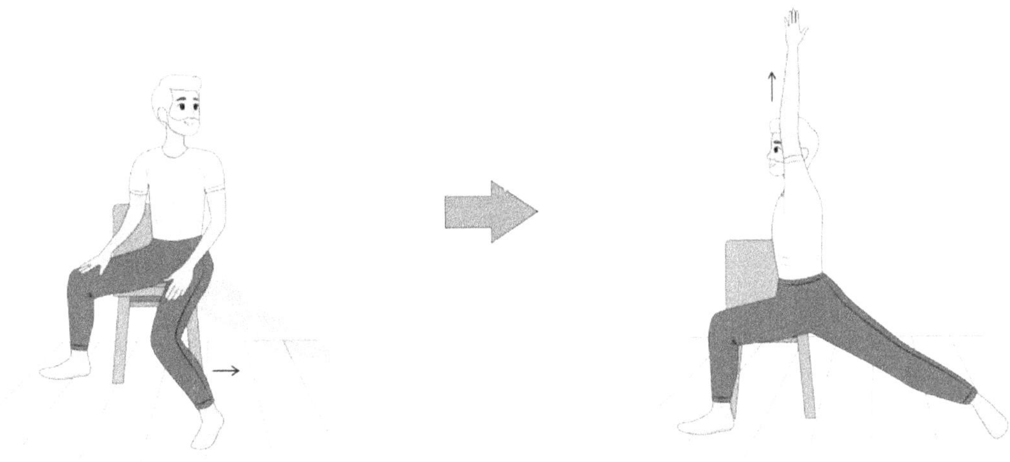

Chair Warrior II:

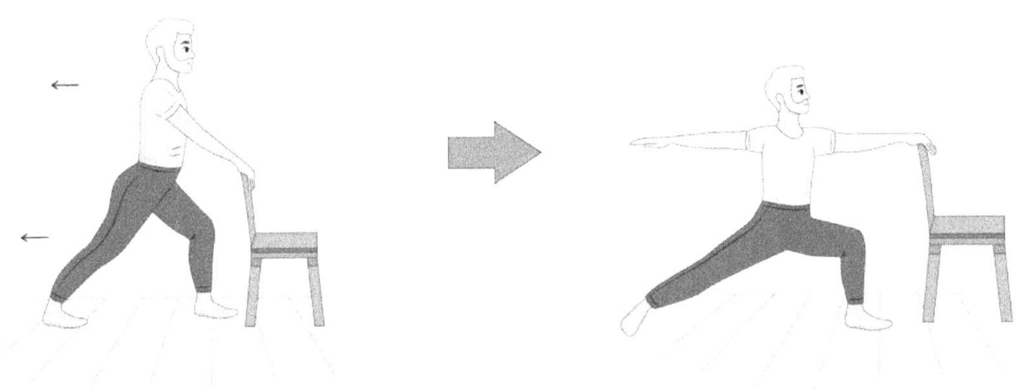

<u>Chair Sun Salutation (Surya Namaskar)</u>

The Chair Sun Salutation, or Surya Namaskar, adapts the dynamic sequence of movements found in traditional Sun Salutations for those who prefer or need to remain seated. This adaptation allows individuals to enjoy the flow and benefits of Surya Namaskar, including improved flexibility, increased circulation and enhanced mental focus from the comfort of a chair. The Chair Sun Salutation offers a comprehensive workout that stimulates the cardiovascular system, stretches the muscles, and calms the mind by incorporating upper body stretches, forward bends, and gentle backbends. It's a holistic exercise that promotes the harmony of body and mind, making it accessible and beneficial for people of all ages and fitness levels. Practicing this modified sequence can build strength in the arms and shoulders, improve spinal flexibility, and foster a more profound sense of inner peace and mindfulness.

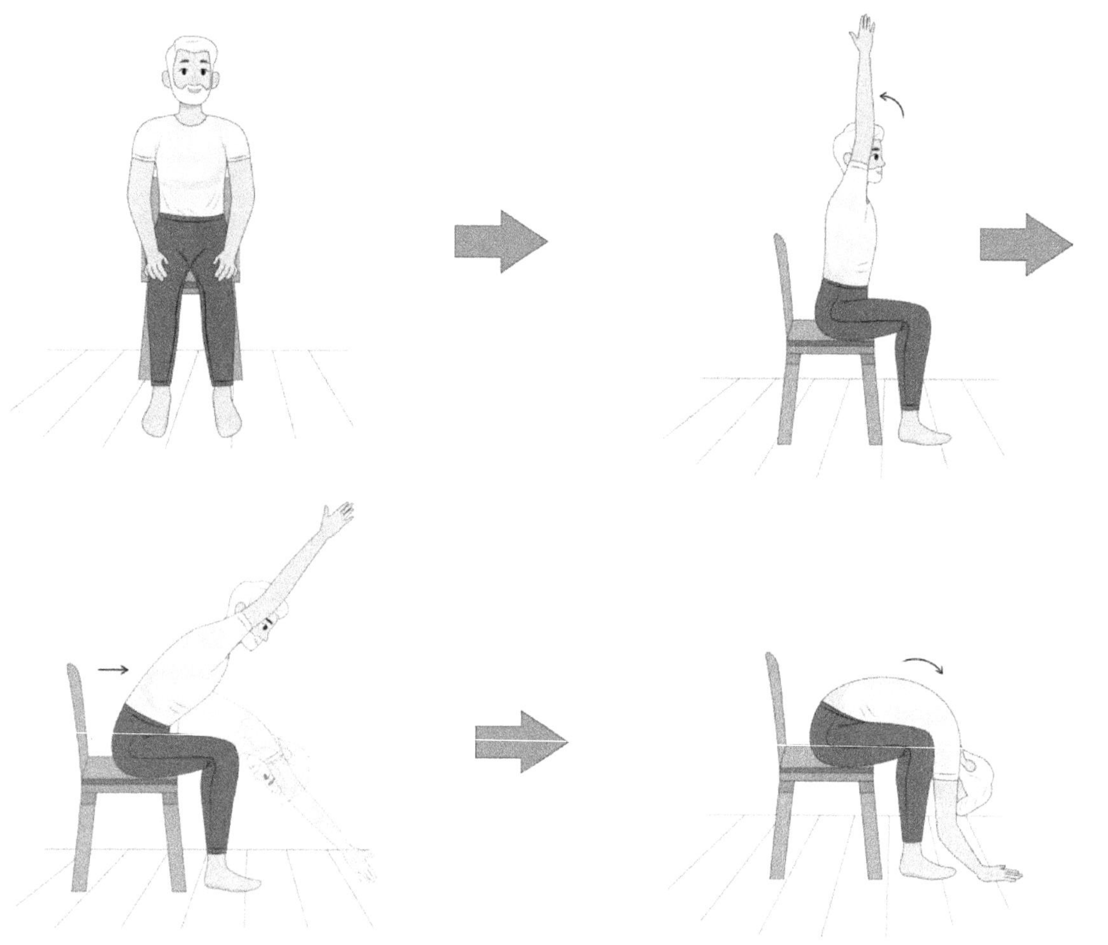

As we transition from the enriching exploration of chair yoga poses to the empowering 28-Day Chair Yoga Challenge, we bridge the gap between learning and practice. The poses we've delved into lay the groundwork for a transformative journey, equipping us with the tools for a more mindful, balanced existence. The upcoming challenge is designed as a series of exercises and a holistic approach to wellness, emphasizing consistency, adaptability, and mindfulness. Engaging daily with the poses, we cultivate a deeper connection to our bodies and minds, fostering growth, flexibility, and strength. This journey invites us to embrace the full potential of chair yoga, ensuring a rewarding experience that transcends the physical enriching our lives profoundly.

Note on Maximizing Results from the 28-Day Chair Yoga Challenge.

Embark on a transformative journey with our 28-Day Chair Yoga Challenge, designed as an exercise routine and a holistic approach to enhancing your health and wellness. This challenge offers a unique opportunity to deepen your connection with body and mind. To ensure the best possible experience, please consider the following guidelines:

Consistency is Key: Commit to practicing daily, even if for brief periods. Regular practice builds strength, flexibility, and a lasting yoga routine.

Listen to Your Body: Acknowledge your current health limitations and adjust accordingly. Yoga is a journey of personal growth and mindful movement, not perfection. Adapt poses to ensure comfort and safety, prioritizing your well-being above all.

The Challenge aims to gently enhance your health and mobility, always considering your body's needs. Join this rewarding journey and experience the transformative effects of chair yoga.

Wishing you a fruitful journey,
Riley Miller

Chapter 6: 28 Days of Challenge Chair Yoga

You will change and feel better when you start the 28-Day Chair Yoga Challenge. The program breaks into four weeks, each building upon the previous one. Each week introduces a different theme to aid your learning and growth.

In Week 1, "Starting a Chair Yoga Adventure," simple poses and gentle moves help you get used to the practice and set you up for more difficult ones.

In Week 2, "Building Flexibility and Strength," you will engage in deeper stretches and strength-building poses to enhance your balance between flexibility and muscle tone.

Week 3 is about "Balance and Coordination," essential for improving your daily life and yoga practice. Using your chair as a support, you'll start doing exercises to test and improve your balance and agility this week.

In the last week, "Deepening Practice and Mindfulness," you build on what you've already learned. It mixes the physical parts of yoga with mindfulness and meditation. This way, you will get stronger and become calmer and more aware.

The Challenge emphasizes daily habits such as mindful foundation exercises, breathing techniques, and visualization. These practices help set the appropriate atmosphere, keeping you present and focused during each session. The program encourages you to engage in these exercises daily for 28 days, fostering greater flexibility in both mind and body.

In 28 days, you'll enjoy improved physical health and a stronger connection with your mind and body, setting a solid foundation for ongoing chair yoga and a broader wellness journey.

The 28-Day Chair Yoga Challenge has structured weekly themes and a thorough weekly planner. This planner is essential for keeping track of your progress, setting daily goals, and thinking about what you learned after each lesson. It's like a personal journal because you can write down the things you do every day, how long you spend on them, and any thoughts or feelings you have. This practice of reflection helps you get more involved with the challenge, which means you'll have a more rewarding and life-changing 28 days.

Establishing Daily Rituals for the Chair Yoga Challenge of 28 Days

Embark on a mindfulness and activities challenge that guides you through each day of the 28-Day Chair Yoga Challenge. Begin your sessions by focusing on breathing techniques and the Seated Mindful Foundation to foster calmness and present-moment awareness. Follow this with stretches and tailored warm-up exercises to ready your body for the upcoming yoga practice. Emphasize the importance of these routines before and after your sessions to enhance your overall experience. Incorporate meditation, visualization, and movement planning into your routine to maximize the benefits of your chair yoga practice.

You must engage in these breathing and mindfulness exercises, warm-ups, and Stretches each day for the 28-day challenge. Consistency is essential to get the most out of chair yoga and improve mental clarity and physical flexibility.

Before Exercises:

Before we dive into our daily chair yoga challenge routines for the next 28 days, let's recall the essential dietary and hydration guidelines from Chapter 2. As we've previously discussed, eating at the right time and with the right foods can help you reap the benefits of your yoga practice. This approach to nutrition and the daily practices you are about to begin will significantly enhance your journey with yoga. Before exercising, give your body enough time to digest food and consume meals that adequately fuel your body.

Seated Mindful Foundation Exercise:

1. **Objective:** This exercise aims to ground you in the present, helping to clear your mind of distractions and stress and preparing you for a focused yoga session.
2. **Preparation:**
- **Chair:** Choose a chair where you can sit comfortably with your feet flat on the floor and your back supported.
- **Environment:** Find a quiet space where you won't be disturbed.
3. **Steps:**
- **Getting Comfortable:** Sit in the middle of the chair with a straight yet relaxed posture. Rest your hands gently on your lap. Place your feet firmly on the ground, establishing a stable hip-width base.
- **Closing Your Eyes and Focusing Inward:** Softly close your eyes to minimize external visual stimuli. Turn your attention inward, away from any external concerns or distractions.
- **Clearing the Mind:** Consciously let go of thoughts about your day, worries, or pending tasks. Imagine your mind as a cluttered room that you're tidying up, putting thoughts away into drawers for later.
- **Breath Awareness:** Focus on your breath. Notice the sensation of air entering through your nostrils, filling your lungs, and then leaving your body.

- Observe the rise and fall of your chest and belly with each breath. This observation helps anchor you in the present moment.
- **Body Sensation and Sound Awareness:** Shift your attention to any sensations in your body, such as relaxation, tension, or even the feel of your clothes against your skin. Please pay attention to the sounds surrounding you, no matter how faint they may be. Engaging in this practice deepens your connection to the present moment.
- **Duration:** Aim to maintain this state of mindfulness for 3 to 5 minutes. This time allows you to transition smoothly into a more meditative state, preparing your mind and body for yoga.

Breathing Exercises for Focus and Relaxation:

Objective: These breathing exercises aim to relax your body, ease your mind, and improve your focus, forming an essential foundation for your yoga practice.

Steps:

- **Diaphragmatic Breathing:**
  How to Do It: Sit up straight but relaxed. Place one hand on your abdomen. Breathe slowly through your nose, aiming to direct the air deep into your belly rather than your chest. Feel your abdomen expand under your hand. Then, gently exhale, allowing your belly to fall.
  Purpose: This breathing technique enhances lung capacity and promotes relaxation by activating the parasympathetic nervous system, often called the "rest and digest" system.

- **Counted Breathing:**
  How to Do It: Transition to counted breathing after getting comfortable with diaphragmatic breathing. Inhale deeply through your nose for a count of four, feeling your abdomen expand. Hold this breath for a count of two. Then, exhale smoothly through your mouth or nose for a count of four, consciously relaxing your body further with each exhale.
  Purpose: This pattern helps regulate your breathing, leading to a better oxygen supply and a calmer mind. It's particularly effective for reducing stress and improving concentration.
  Duration: Spend approximately 3 to 5 minutes on these exercises. Begin with diaphragmatic breathing to establish a rhythm, then incorporate counted breathing to deepen your focus and relaxation.
  Closing Thought: By dedicating time to these preparatory exercises, you're enhancing your physical readiness for yoga and cultivating a mental space conducive to a more profound and impactful practice.

Warm-up exercises and Stretches

After finishing the "Seated Mindful Foundation and Breathing Exercises," **it's essential to do some warm-up moves and stretches**. These warm-ups are just for chair yoga and help prepare your body for more yoga. They make you less likely to get hurt and improve your yoga. Going on to the next steps is a crucial part of chair yoga. It brings together mind exercises and physical activity for your overall health.

1. Introduction and Setting (1 Minute): Find a comfortable position. Sit on your chair, feet flat on the ground, hands resting on your lap. Take a moment to relax your shoulders and take several deep breaths.

Gentle Neck Stretches:

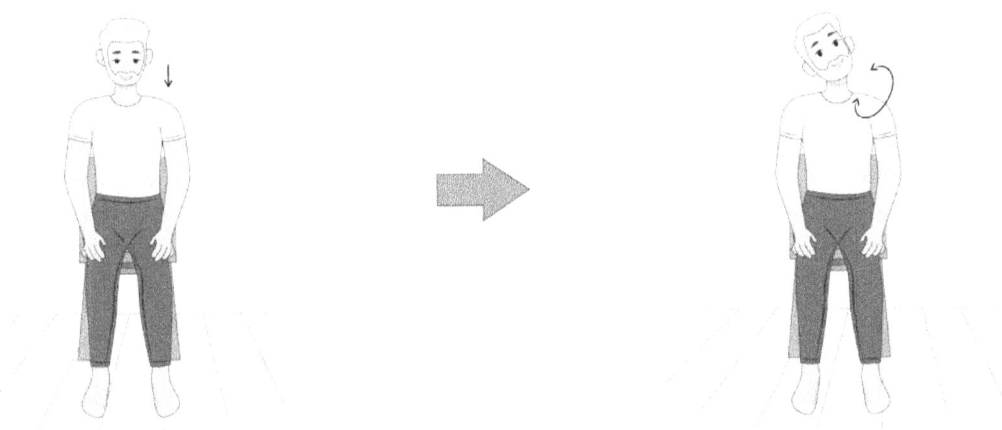

1.Begin by gently lowering your chin towards your chest to initiate the neck's circular motion.

• Ensure your movements are slow and mindful to maintain comfort.

2. Gradually roll your head to the right, aiming to bring your right ear towards your right shoulder without lifting the shoulder.

3. Continue the motion by gently tilting your head back, then moving to bring your left ear towards your left shoulder.

• Complete the circle by returning your chin to your chest.

Repetition: Perform this circular movement thrice, reverse the direction, and repeat.

Caution:

• Keep the circles small and controlled to avoid any strain on the neck.

• Move slowly to prevent any dizziness or discomfort.

2. Shoulder and Arm Warm-Up:

Shoulder Rolls:

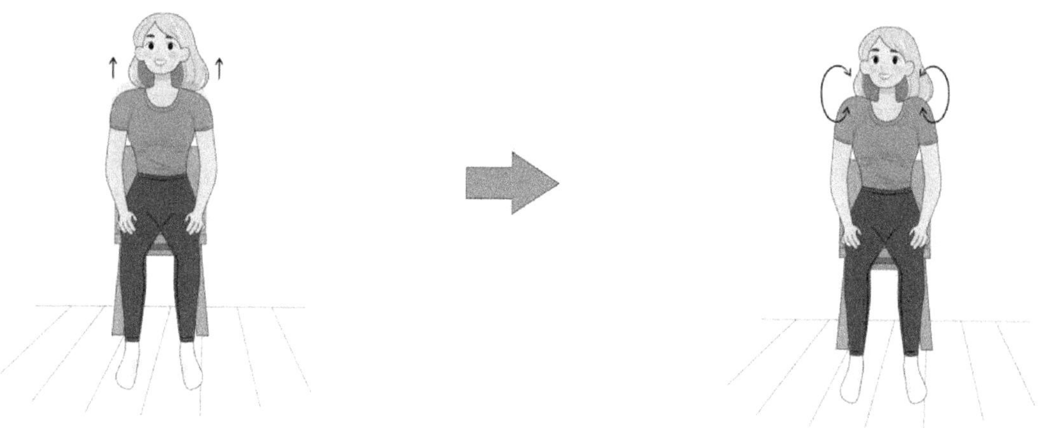

1. Inhale deeply, lifting your shoulders towards your ears.

● Ensure your neck remains long and relaxed.

2. As you exhale, roll your shoulders back, drawing the shoulder blades together, then continue the motion, lowering your shoulders.

● Imagine drawing a circle with your shoulders to encourage full mobility.

Repetition: Perform the forward and backward rolls for 20 seconds each.

Caution:

● Perform the movements gently to avoid any strain.

● Keep the motion controlled, especially if you have any shoulder discomfort.

Arm Stretches:

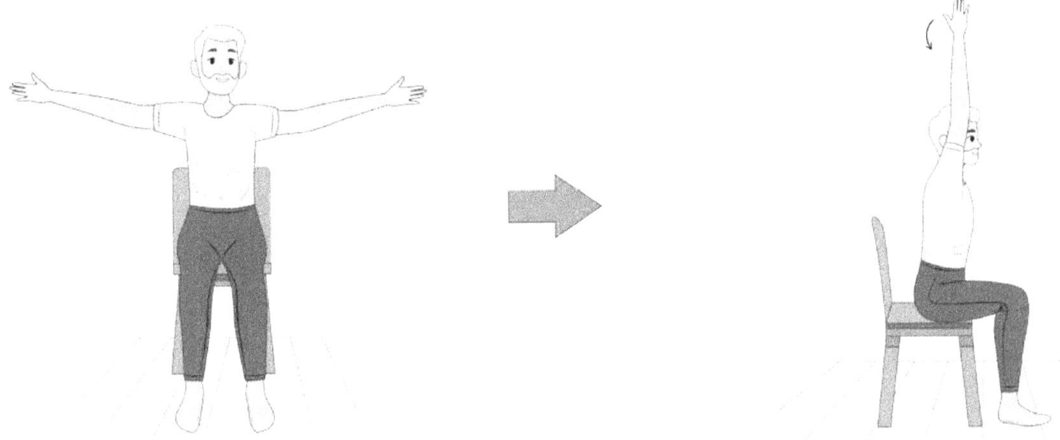

1. Extend your arms to the sides, ensuring they align with your shoulders.

• Keep your shoulders relaxed and down, away from your ears.

2. Slowly raise your arms above your head, keeping them straight as if reaching for the ceiling.

• Imagine stretching the sides of your body to create space between your ribs and hips.

3. Hold this position for a few seconds, focusing on the stretch throughout your upper body. Then, gradually lower your arms back to the starting side position.

Repetition: Repeat this stretching sequence, concentrating on lengthening and relaxing your body.

Caution:

• Move your arms smoothly to avoid any jerky movements or strain.
• Ensure your movements are controlled and aligned with your body's natural range of motion.

Seated Side Stretches

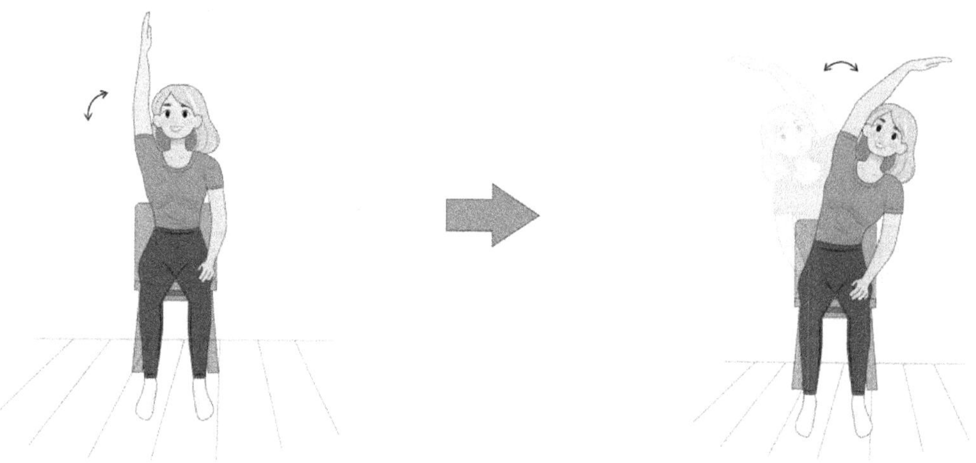

1. Sit upright and raise your right arm overhead. Inhale deeply.

2. As you exhale, gently lean to the left, stretching the right side of your torso. Keep your left hand on the chair seat for support.

• Ensure both sit bones remain in contact with the seat to maintain balance.

Repetition: Hold the stretch for five deep breaths, then switch sides, stretching the left side of your torso.

Caution: Do not overextend; the goal is a gentle stretch along the side of your body.

Seated Twists:

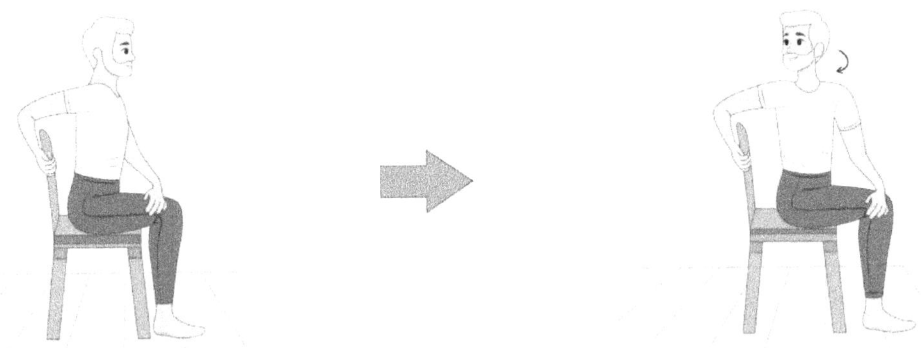

1. Place your right hand on the back of the chair for stability. Take a deep inhalation to prepare.

2. As you exhale, gently rotate your torso to the right, applying gentle pressure with your left hand on your right knee to aid the twist.

- Ensure the twist initiates from the base of your spine, moving upwards.

Repetition: Hold the position on each side for a few seconds, breathing deeply and focusing on the stretch in your spine

Caution:

- Avoid over-twisting; keep the movement gentle and controlled.
- Ensure your feet remain firmly on the ground to maintain balance.

4. Leg and Ankle Mobility:

Leg Extensions

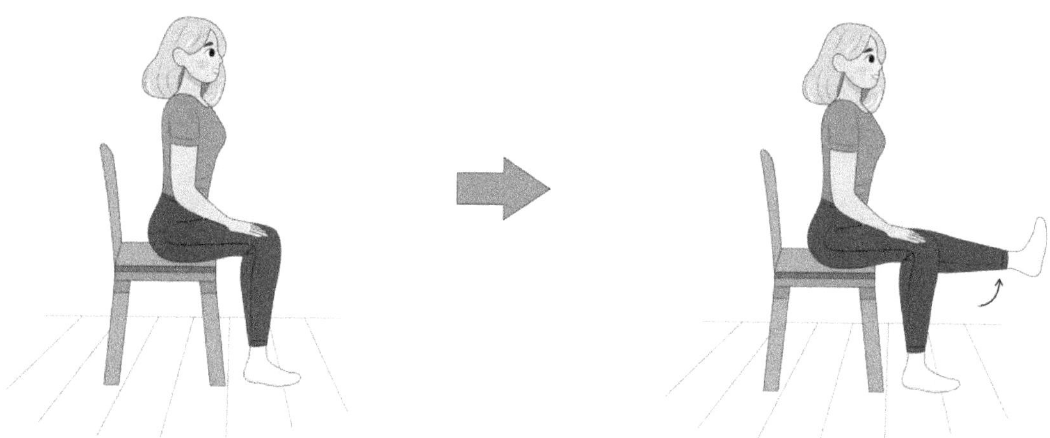

1. Extend one leg straight before you, aiming to keep it parallel to the floor.

● Engage your thigh muscles to maintain the extension.

2. Hold the position for three breaths, focusing on balance and the engagement of your leg muscles.

● Lower the leg gently and switch to the other leg, repeating the extension.

Repetition: Hold each leg for three breaths.

Caution: Ensure you maintain an upright posture to avoid straining your back.

Ankle Rotations

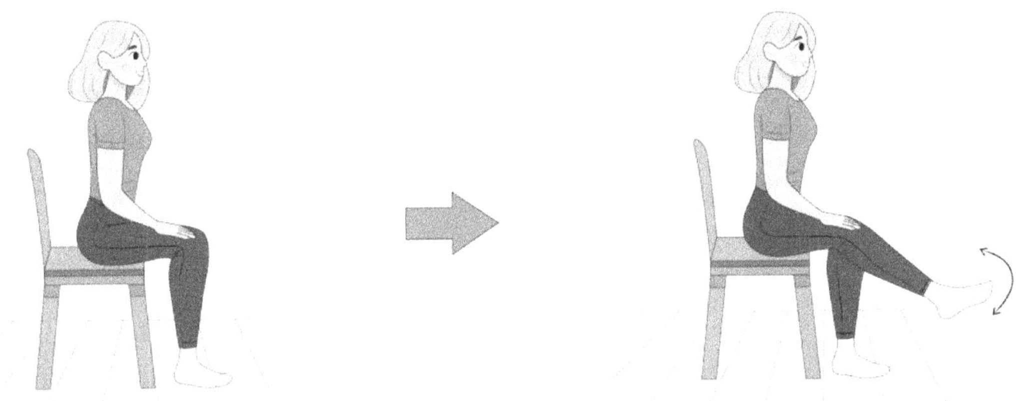

1. Extend one leg on half straight before you.

● Engage your thigh muscles to maintain the extension.

2. Begin by rotating the ankle of the extended leg in a clockwise direction. Aim for five full circles, ensuring the movement originates from the ankle.

● Keep the rest of the leg as still as possible to isolate the movement to the ankle.

3. After completing the clockwise rotations, switch directions to rotate the ankle counterclockwise for another five rotations.

● Focus on making smooth, controlled circles.

Repetition: Complete five rotations in each direction for each ankle.

Caution:

● Ensure that the rotations are slow and controlled to avoid any strain.

● Keep the extended leg still to focus the movement on the ankle.

Remember that these workouts should be comfortable and never painful. If any movement produces discomfort, ease off or avoid it. This 4-minute warm-up activity will gently prepare your body for the chair yoga session, increasing flexibility and assuring a safe and comfortable experience.

Meditation and Visualization Post-Practice

Conclude your chair yoga session with a guided imagery or visualization exercise. Envision a serene environment, such as a tranquil beach or a peaceful forest, engaging all senses to immerse in the calmness. Focus on the serene visuals or shift attention to your breathing, anchoring yourself in peace through each breath's rhythm. This powerful meditation and visualization blend aids in unwinding and achieving mental clarity post-exercise.

Integrating Mindful Movements

After yoga, transition to intentional movement coordination, aligning each motion with your breath for fluidity between poses. This synchronization enhances body-mind connection, balance, and grace, culminating in a mindful and integrated practice, fostering inner peace.

Duration for Optimal Benefits

During the 28-day challenge, aim for 5-10 minutes of mindfulness and breathing exercises before and after yoga. Starting with 3-5 minutes is beneficial, but extending to 5-10 minutes enhances relaxation, the mind-body connection, and the overall experience. This duration is crucial for experiencing the full transformative effect.

Importance of Daily Warm-Ups

Daily warm-up exercises are vital for the 28-day chair yoga challenge, enhancing flexibility and energy and reducing injury risk. These warm-ups are integral to your practice, preparing you physically and mentally for daily activities.

The 28-Day Challenge Planner

This planner section aims to assist you in systematically documenting your chair yoga journey. Daily, record your yoga sessions, establish weekly goals, and jot down your progress and feelings after each practice. This structured approach strengthens your dedication and enhances the benefits of the Challenge.

In the notes area, you have the freedom to detail:

Dates: Keep a record of your practice days.

Moods: Share insights into your emotional state if you wish.

Feelings: Describe any specific emotions or physical sensations experienced during your sessions.

Personal Observations: Jot down any additional thoughts or discoveries you want to remember.

This planner is a personal tool for tracing your 28-day journey, deepening your connection to the practice. Let it be a companion as you navigate your chair yoga adventure, encouraging reflection and growth.

Week 1 Planner

Day	Routine	Goal	Time Spent	Notes
Day 1	Simple Seated Poses and Gentle Shoulder and Back Stretches	Get acquainted with basic motions		
Day 2	Adding Arm Stretches, Exploring Breath Awareness	Improve flexibility and breathing		
Day 3	Intro to Leg Stretches, Continued Breath Work	Enhance leg flexibility and deepen breath awareness		
Day 4	Combining Upper and Lower Body Stretches	Integrate full-body movement		
Day 5	Introduction to Seated Twists and Side Bends	Increase spinal mobility		
Day 6	The Practice of Full Routine Learned So Far	Consolidate learned poses		
Day 7	Rest or Gentle Practice, Reflecting on the Week	Reflect on progress and experiences		

Week 1: Starting a Chair Yoga Adventure

Welcome to the first week of your Chair Yoga journey. This week is about slowly introducing you to chair yoga by focusing on simple poses and moves that are great for beginners. We will learn about different parts of chair yoga daily, starting with basic poses and adding more things over time, like leg moves, arm stretches, and breath work. The goal is to feel comfortable with the basic moves and understand how these workouts can help you become more flexible, stronger, and smarter. Remember that this starts a long journey to better health and well-being. Let's begin this trip with a ready heart and an open mind.

Day 1: Introduction to Chair Yoga and Gentle Upper Body Stretching

Preparation: Begin with a 3-5 minute seated mindfulness and deep breathing exercise session. This initial phase sets the foundation, calms the mind, and readies the body for the following stretches. Don't forget to do warm-up exercises before your exercise program, as outlined in Chapter 5

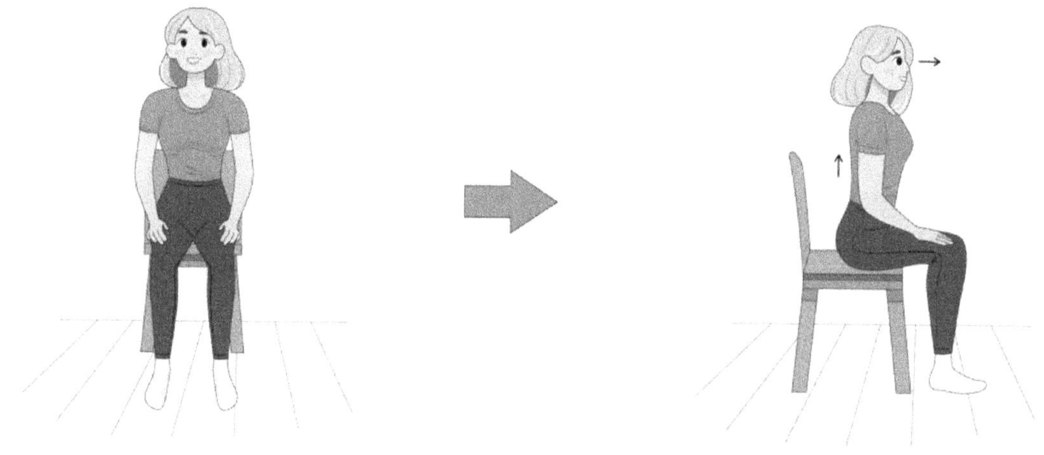

Objective: The aim is to relieve tension in the back and shoulders

1) Seated Mountain Pose (Tadasana):

1. Sit with your back straight, feet flat on the ground, and hands resting on your thighs.

2. Exhale, gently relaxing your shoulders down away from your ears.

3. Maintain this posture for five deep breaths, concentrating on a tall, stable posture.

Caution:

- Do not arch your back or elevate your shoulders, as this can compromise the stability of the pose.
- Focus on maintaining an even distribution of weight across your sit bones.

2) Seated Cat-Cow:

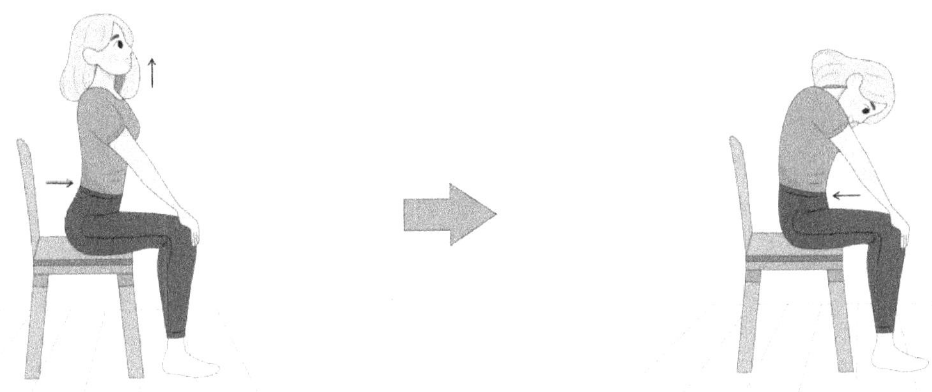

1. Sit on the edge of a chair with your feet firmly planted and your hands on your knees.

2. Begin by gently arching your back and tilting your head slightly to open your chest.

- Breathe in deeply as you arch.

3. Transition to rounding your back, bringing your chin to your chest, and pulling your belly inward.

- Exhale slowly during this movement.

4. Flow between the arching and rounding movements with each breath, focusing on smooth transitions to enhance spinal flexibility.

Repetition: Perform this sequence five times.

Caution: Ensure movements are gentle to avoid back strain.

3. Shoulder Rolls:

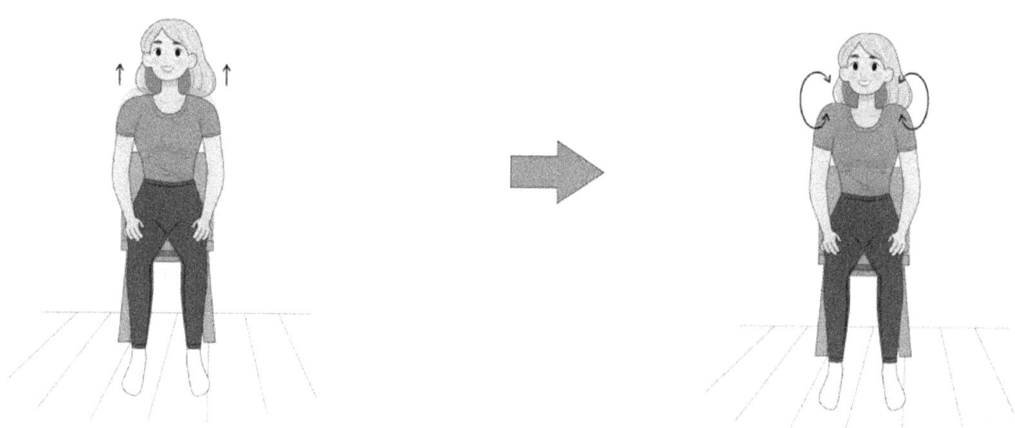

1. Inhale deeply, lifting your shoulders towards your ears.

- Ensure your neck remains long and relaxed.

2. As you exhale, roll your shoulders back, drawing the shoulder blades together, then continue the motion, lowering your shoulders.

- Imagine drawing a circle with your shoulders to encourage full mobility.

3. Reverse the direction, rolling your shoulders forward for another 20 seconds to balance the movement.

Repetition: Perform the forward and backward rolls for 20 seconds each.

Caution:

- Perform the movements gently to avoid any strain.
- Keep the motion controlled, especially if you have any shoulder discomfort.

After Exercises: Following the exercises, engage in visualization and meditation, then Coordination of Intentional Movements as described in the subchapter Establishing Daily Rituals for the Chair Yoga Challenge of 28 Days in Chapter 6.

Day 2: Adding Arm Stretches, Exploring Breath Awareness

Goal: Improve flexibility and breathing

Before Exercises: Do mindful foundation breathing exercises, then warm up and stretches

DAY 2

EXERCISE	SETS
☐ Side Stretch	3 brs/side
☐ Arm Stretch	3 brs/arm
☐ Cat-Cow	x5

1) Seated Side Stretch

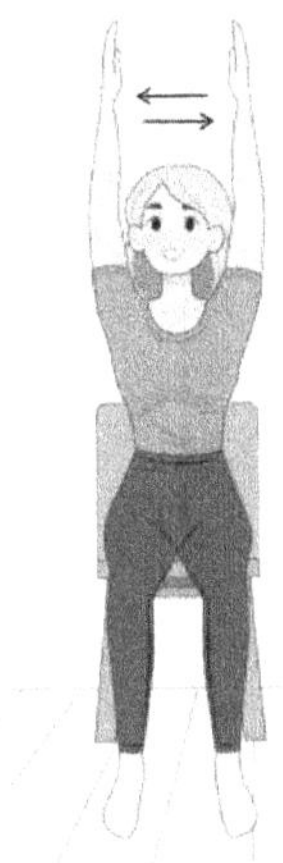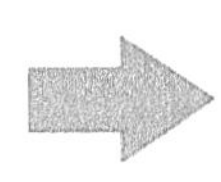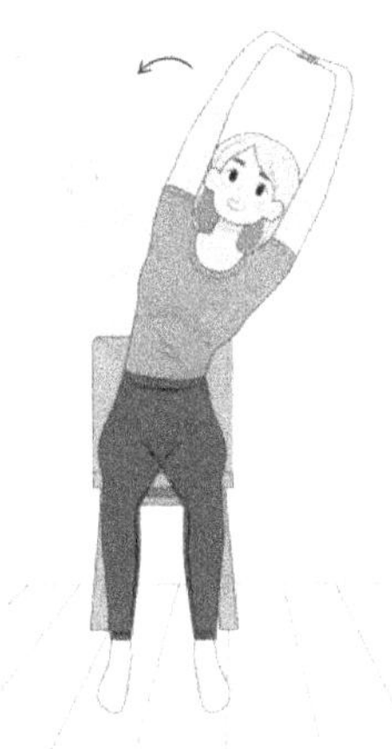

1. Sit straight, arms extended overhead, fingers interlaced.

- Take a deep breath in, stretching your spine upwards.

2. As you exhale, lean to one side, maintaining equal pressure on both sit bones to keep the stretch balanced.

- Ensure both sit bones remain in contact with the seat.

3. Hold this position for three deep breaths, feeling the stretch along your side.

4. Inhale as you return to the center, then switch sides, repeating the stretch.

Repetition: Hold for three breaths on each side.

Caution: Ensure not to lean forward or backward; the movement is strictly sideways.

2) Arm Cross Stretch:

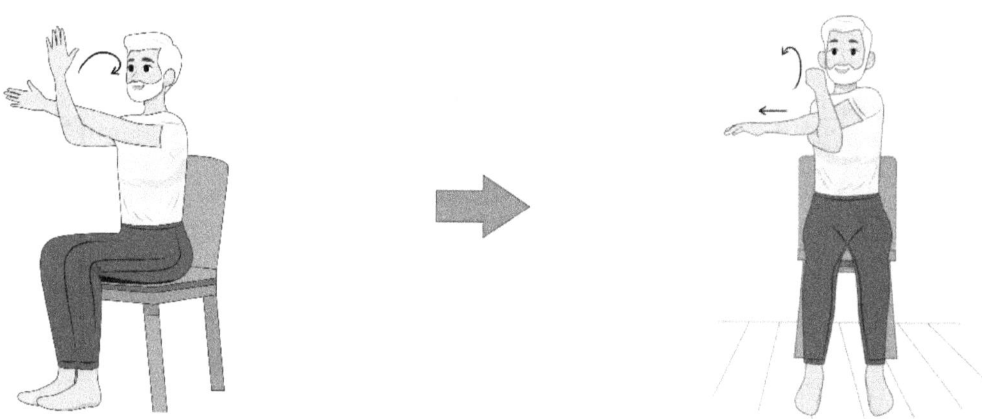

1. Sit, feet flat, arms by your side.

2. Extend one arm straight across your body at chest level.

• Keep your extended arm parallel to the ground.

3. Use the opposite hand to gently press against the outside of the stretching arm, near the elbow, to deepen the stretch.

• Ensure your shoulders remain low and relaxed, avoiding any shrugging.

4. Take three deep breaths, focusing on the stretch across your shoulder and upper arm.

5. Slowly release and switch arms, repeating the stretch on the other side.

Repetition: Perform the stretch three times on each arm.

Caution:

- Do not apply too much pressure; the aim is a gentle, relieving stretch.
- Maintain a relaxed posture to prevent any unnecessary tension.

3) Seated Cat-Cow:

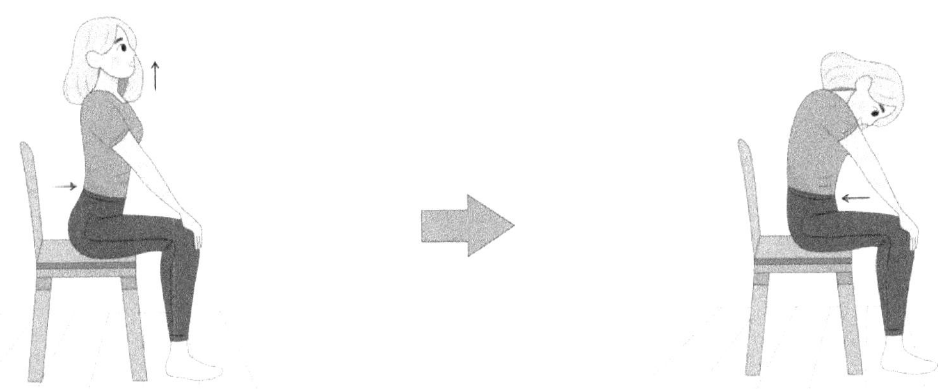

1. Sit on the edge of a chair with your feet firmly planted and your hands on your knees.

2. Begin by gently arching your back and tilting your head slightly to open your chest.

- Breathe in deeply as you arch.

3. Transition to rounding your back, bringing your chin to your chest, and pulling your belly inward.

- Exhale slowly during this movement.

4. Flow between the arching and rounding movements with each breath, focusing on smooth transitions to enhance spinal flexibility.

Repetition: Perform this sequence five times.

After Exercises: Following the exercises, engage in visualization and meditation, then Coordination of Intentional Movements.

Day 3: Intro to Leg Stretches, Continued Breath Work

Goal: Enhance leg flexibility and deepen breath awareness

Before Exercises: Follow the same routine as Day 1

DAY 3		
	EXERCISE	**SETS**
☐	Forward Bend	3 brs
☐	Leg Lifts	3 brs/leg
☐	Ankle Rotations	x5/side

1) Gentle Seated Forward Bend:

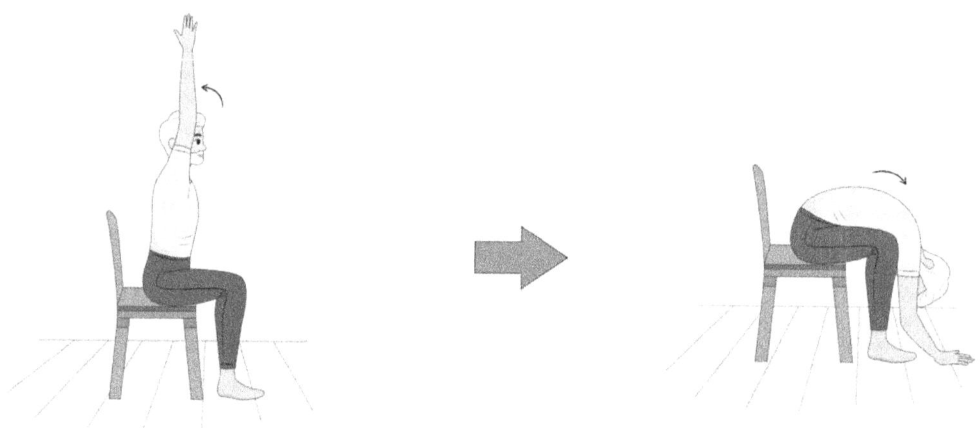

1. Sit straight. Arms extended overhead
2. Inhale deeply, then gently lean forward from your hips as you exhale, reaching towards your feet.

3. Focus on maintaining a straight back as much as possible to deepen the stretch along your spine and hamstrings.

Repetition: Stay in this position for three full breaths, gently increasing the stretch with each exhale.

Caution: Keep the stretch gentle, and avoid overstretching or jerky movements.

2) Seated Leg Lifts:

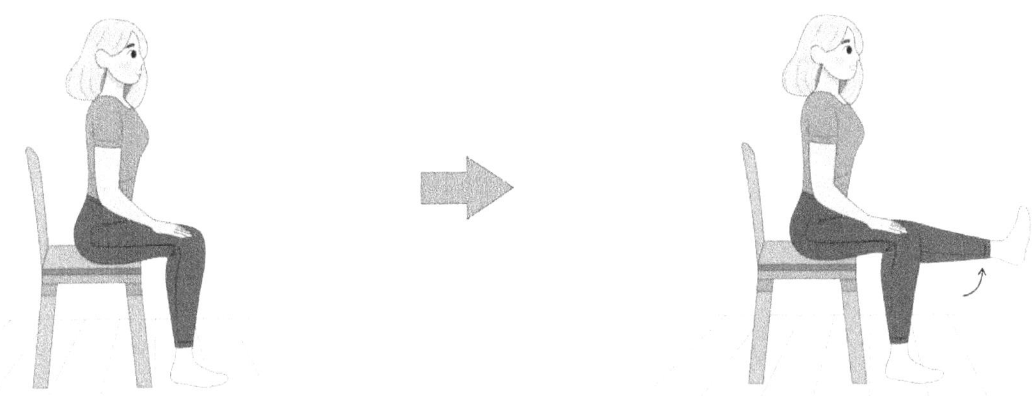

1. Extend one leg straight before you, aiming to keep it parallel to the floor.

- Engage your thigh muscles to maintain the extension.

2. Hold the position for three breaths, focusing on balance and the engagement of your leg muscles.

3. Lower the leg gently and switch to the other leg, repeating the extension.

Repetition: Hold each leg for three breaths.

Caution:

- Ensure you maintain an upright posture to avoid straining your back.

Ankle Rotations

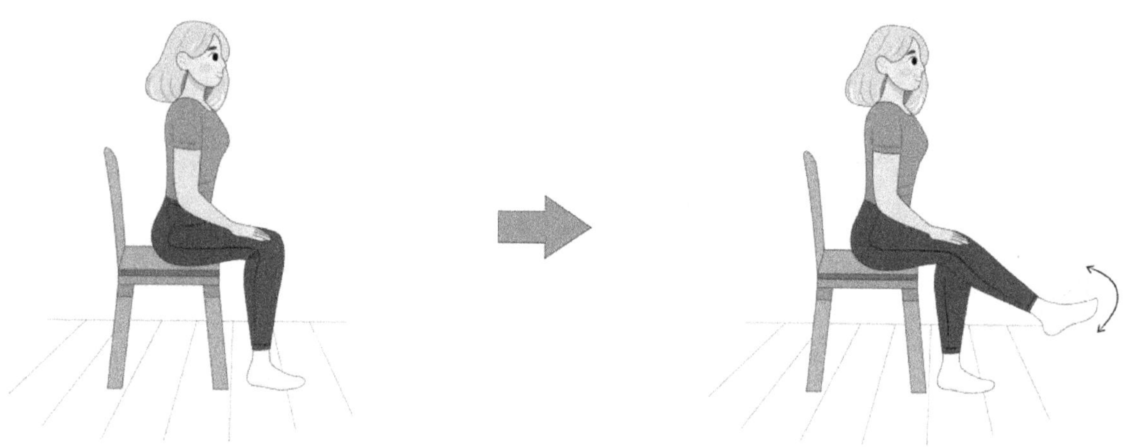

1. Extend one leg half-straight before you

- Engage your thigh muscles to maintain the extension.

2. Begin by rotating the ankle of the extended leg in a clockwise direction. Aim for five full circles, ensuring the movement originates from the ankle.

- Keep the rest of the leg as still as possible to isolate the movement to the ankle.

3. After completing the clockwise rotations, switch directions to rotate the ankle counterclockwise for another five rotations.

- Focus on making smooth, controlled circles.

Repetition: Complete five rotations in each direction for each ankle.

Caution:

- Ensure that the rotations are slow and controlled to avoid any strain.
- Keep the extended leg still to focus the movement on the ankle.

Day 4: Combining Upper and Lower Body Stretches

Goal: Integrate full-body movement

Before Exercises: As in previous days

DAY 4

EXERCISE	SETS
☐ Seated Twist	3 brs/side
☐ Chair Pigeon	3 brs/side
☐ Eagle Arms	3 brs/side

1) Seated Twist:

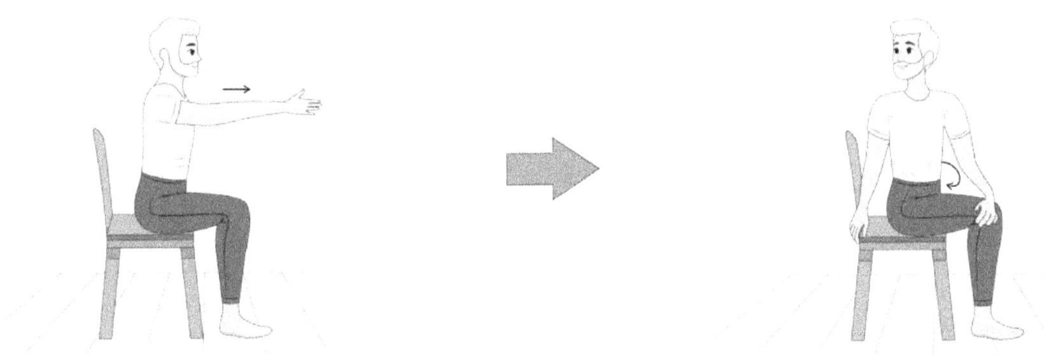

1. Sit firmly on the chair, ensuring an upright posture
2. Inhale deeply, lifting your arms to shoulder height, focusing on engaging your core.
- Visualize lengthening your spine with the inhalation

3. As you exhale, twist your torso to the right, placing your left hand on your right knee for leverage and your right hand behind you for support.
- Imagine wringing out tension from your spine with the exhalation.

4. Maintain the twist, keeping your spine elongated, and gaze over your right shoulder for three deep breaths.

Repetition: Inhale to return to the center with arms raised, then exhale as you repeat the twist to the left side. Perform three deep breaths on each side.

Caution: Begin the twist from your lower back, progressing upwards; avoid neck strain by keeping the movement smooth.

2) Seated Chair Pigeon:

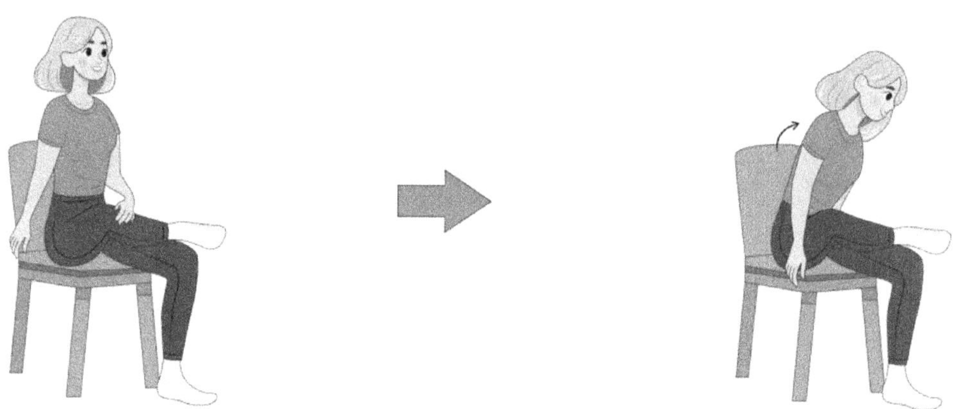

1. Sit with legs uncrossed, maintaining a straight spine.

2. Gently lift your right ankle, placing it on your left knee and allowing the right knee to open to the side.

● Flex your foot to protect your knee.

3. Inhale to prepare, exhale as you lean forward slightly, hinging at the hips to deepen your right hip and glute stretch.

● Keep your back flat, imagining a string pulling you forward from your chest.

Repetition: Slowly return to an upright position and switch to stretch the other side. Hold for three breaths on each side.

Caution: Move into the stretch gently to avoid overextending the hip or placing undue pressure on the knee.

3) Seated Eagle Arms:

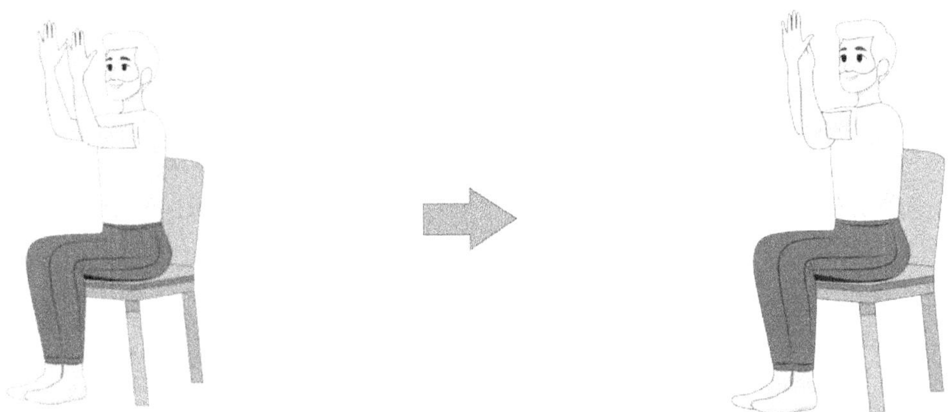

1. Sit upright with feet flat on the ground and arms extended.

2. Extend your arms forward, crossing the right arm over the left at the elbows.

3. Bend your elbows upwards, then wrap your forearms so your palms meet, or grab onto the opposite shoulder if the palms don't reach.

● Envision drawing energy into your core as you lift your elbows.

4. Maintain this wrapped position, focusing on the stretch across the back of your shoulders for three breaths.

Repetition: Unwrap and gently shake your arms before switching the cross to the other side. Hold for three breaths on each side.

Caution: Keep your shoulders relaxed, focusing on the stretch rather than the depth of the arm wrap.

After Exercises: Continue as in Day 1.

Day 5: Introduction to Seated Twists and Side Bends

Goal: Increase spinal mobility

Before Exercises: As in Day 1

DAY 5

EXERCISE	SETS
☐ Side Bend	5 brs/side
☐ Spinal Twist	3 brs/side
☐ Neck Stretch	3 brs/side

1) Dynamic Seated Side Bend:

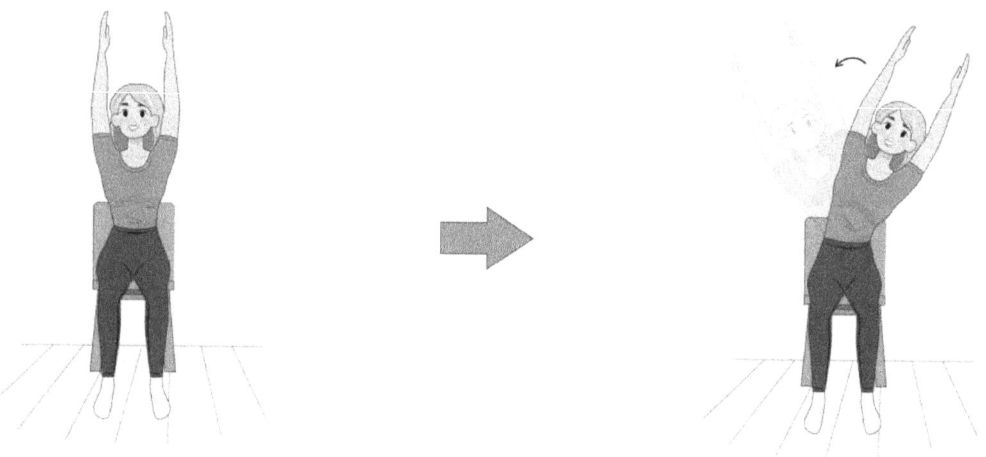

1. Begin seated with your spine straight, arms reaching overhead. Inhale deeply to prepare, elongating your spine.

● As you exhale, lean to one side, keeping your arms extended. Imagine stretching over a ball to maintain the arc of your body.

2. Smoothly transition to the other side, creating a flowing side-to-side movement.

● Focus on the stretch along your side of the body, ensuring even distribution of the movement.

Repetition: Continue this motion for five breaths, alternating sides with each exhale.

Caution:

● Maintain a tall spine to enhance the stretch and prevent compression.
● Ensure movements are fluid, avoiding any sharp or jerky motions.

2) Gentle Seated Spinal Twist:

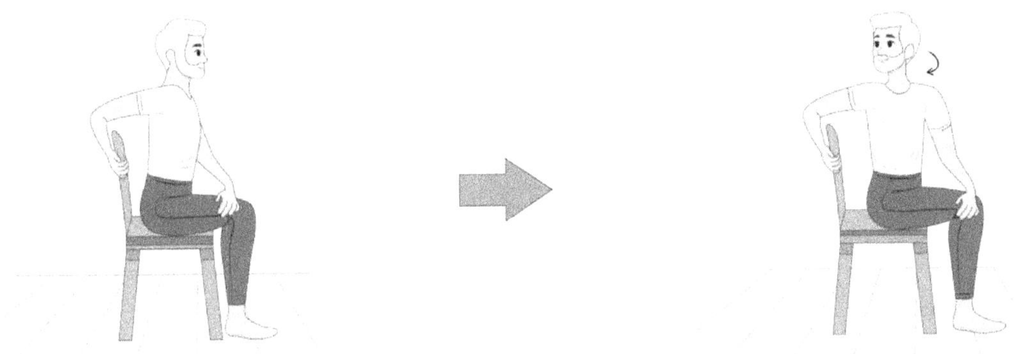

1. Sit has feet flat and is tall. Inhale to lengthen further.

- Engage your core lightly to support the spine.

2. Exhale, gently twisting to one side. Use your hands for light leverage, not force.

- Focus on the sensation of the twist, allowing it to progress naturally.

Repetition: Hold for three breaths, experiencing the stretch and twist in your spine. Inhale back to center and switch sides, ensuring a balanced approach.

Caution:

- The wist should originate from the lower back, progressing upward.
- Avoid over-twisting or straining the neck.

3) Seated Lateral Neck Stretch:

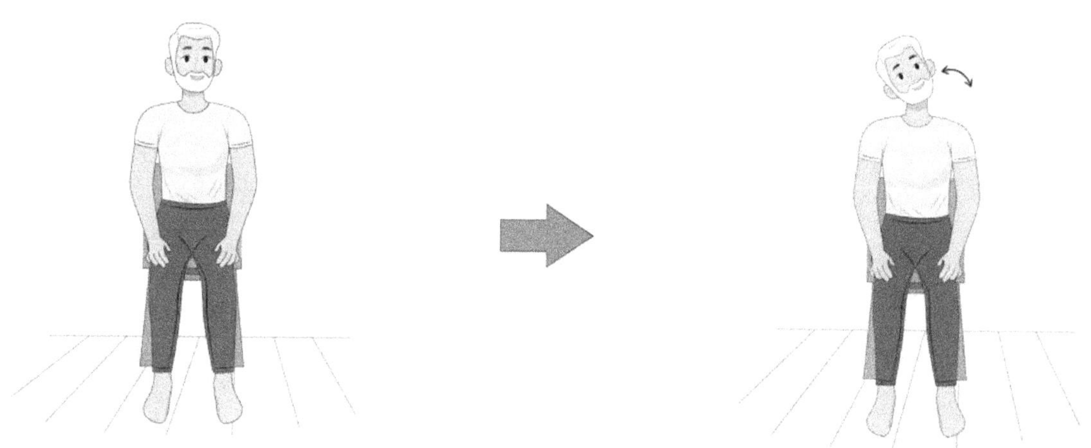

1. Sit upright, shoulders down. Tilt your head to one side, aiming for a gentle ear-to-shoulder stretch.

- Breathe deeply, allowing the stretch to deepen naturally with each exhale.

2. Maintain the tilt for three breaths, focusing on the stretch along the opposite side of your neck.

3. Carefully return to the center and repeat on the opposite side for symmetry.

Repetition: Repeat the stretch, taking three deep breaths per side.

Caution:

- Ensure the shoulder opposite the tilt remains relaxed and lowered.
- Adjust the intensity of the stretch to avoid discomfort.

After Exercises: Follow the same closing routine as earlier days.

Day 6: Practice of Full Routine Learned So Far

DAY 6

Goal: Consolidate learned poses

Before Exercises: As in previous days.

EXERCISE	SETS
☐ CONSOLIDATE	as in
☐ LEARNED	previous
☐ POSES	times

Routine:

Perform a sequence of selected exercises from Days 1-5, transitioning smoothly from one pose to the next.

After Exercises: Follow the same closing routine as earlier days.

Day 7: Rest or Gentle Practice, Reflecting on the Week

DAY 7

Goal: Reflect on progress and experiences

Before Exercises: As in previous days.

EXERCISE	SETS
☐ Revisits the most	as in
☐ beneficial poses	previous
☐ from the week	days

Routine:

Choose to rest or engage in a gentle practice that revisits the most beneficial poses from the week.

Focus on reflection and how your body feels after a week of practice

After Exercises: Follow the same closing routine as earlier days.

Week 2: Building Flexibility and Strength

As we begin Week 2 of our Chair Yoga program, let's take a moment to review the fundamental techniques we learned in Week 1 using easy, beginner-friendly poses. Using this foundation as a starting point, we now concentrate on improving our strength and flexibility with more challenging workouts. This week, focus on developing your practice with various routines to help you consistently improve. Remember to consider your everyday experiences and acknowledge your progress in strength, flexibility, and general well-being as we explore these new dimensions. Accept this chance to develop and enhance your chair yoga practice as we go forward on our path.

Week 2 Planner

Day	Routine	Goal	Time Spent	Notes
Day 8	Strength-focused Chair Yoga Poses	Build core and upper body strength		
Day 9	Enhancing Flexibility with Deeper Stretches	Improve overall flexibility		
Day 10	Integration of Strength and Flexibility Poses	Balance strength and flexibility		
Day 11	Seated and Standing Poses Combination	Enhance coordination and strength		
Day 12	Focused Breathing with Movement	Synchronize breath with movements		
Day 13	Advanced Seated Twists and Side Bends	Deepen spinal stretches		
Day 14	Review of Week's Poses and Techniques	Consolidate learning from the week		

Day 8: Strength-focused Chair Yoga Poses

DAY 8

Goal: Build core and upper body strength.

Before Exercises: As in previous days.

EXERCISE	SETS
☐ Chair Plank:	5 breaths
☐ Leg Lifts	x5/leg
☐ Warrior I	5 brs/side

1) Chair Plank

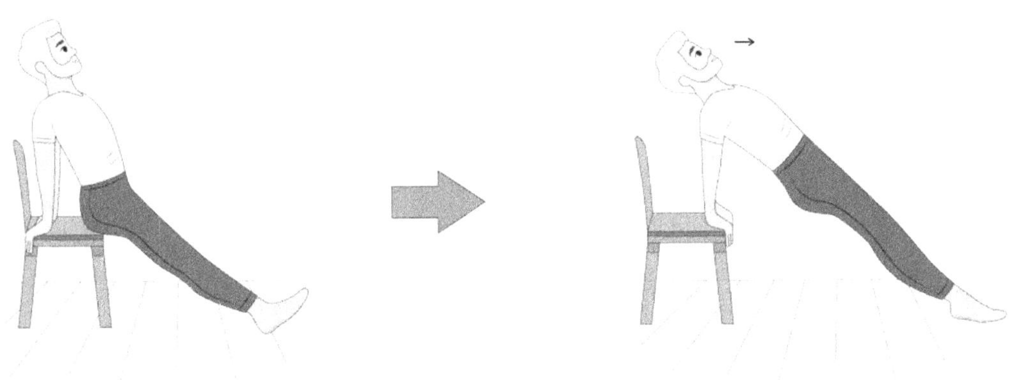

1. Start sitting at the chair's edge, firmly placing your hands on the sides.

● Ensure your feet are together, extending straight in front of you.

2. Press down through your hands, engage your core, and lift your hips to bring your body into a straight line from shoulders to heels.

● Focus on creating a straight line, avoiding sagging or lifting the hips too high.

Repetition: Hold this plank position for five deep breaths, focusing on steady breathing

Caution:
● Check the chair's stability before beginning.
● Keep your body straight to avoid strain on your lower back.

2) Seated Leg Lifts:

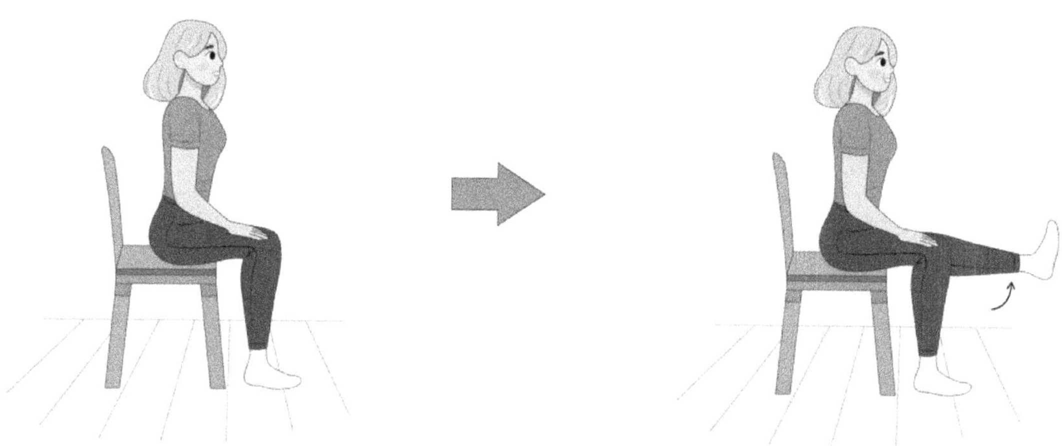

1. Extend one leg straight before you, aiming to keep it parallel to the floor.

• Engage your thigh muscles to maintain the extension.

2. Hold the position for three breaths, focusing on balance and the engagement of your leg muscles.

3. Lower the leg gently and switch to the other leg, repeating the extension.

Repetition: Perform five lifts per leg.

Caution: Ensure movements are slow and controlled to maintain balance and prevent sudden jerks.

3) Chair Warrior I:

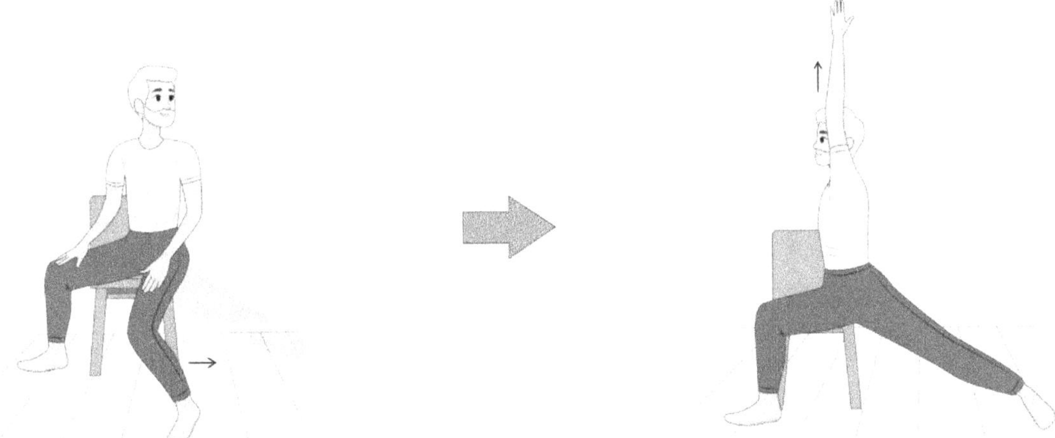

1. Sit on the edge of a chair, facing forward. Place your feet flat on the ground.

2. Extend your right leg back, resting the ball of the foot on the floor and keeping your left foot facing forward.

● Ensure your left knee is directly above your ankle, not extending past your toes.

3. Rotate your torso to face the front of the chair, aligning your hips forward.

● Keep your back straight and chest lifted.

4. Raise your arms overhead, palms facing each other or touching.

● Shoulders should be relaxed, not hunched up to your ears.

5. Look forward or slightly up, maintaining a steady gaze.

● Ensure your breathing is even and steady; do not hold your breath.

Repetition: Hold for five deep breaths, then switch sides.

Caution: Monitor your front knee to ensure it does not extend past your toes, protecting the knee joint.

After Exercises: Following the exercises, engage in visualization and meditation, then Coordination of Intentional Movements.

Day 9: Enhancing Flexibility with Deeper Stretches

Goal: Improve overall flexibility.

Before Exercises: As in previous days.

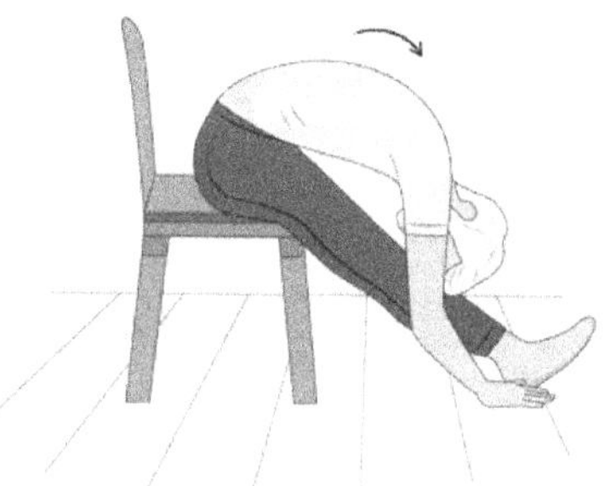

1) Seated Forward Bend:

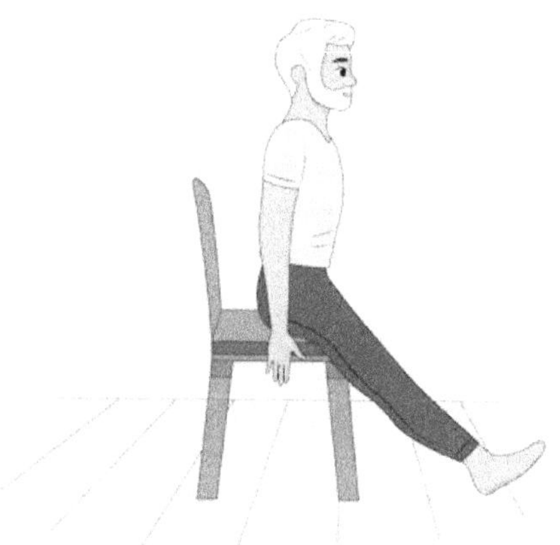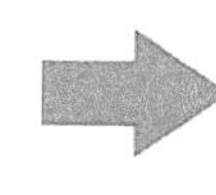

1. Start with your legs extended and your spine tall. Inhale to prepare, focusing on lengthening your spine upwards.

● As you exhale, hinge forward from the hips, aiming to keep your back straight to target the stretch in the hamstrings.

2. Reach towards your toes, keeping the stretch comfortable and within your range of motion.

● Allow each exhale to deepen the stretch gently, focusing on relaxation and flexibility.

Repetition: Hold for five breaths.

Caution: Avoid rounding the back to prevent strain.

2) Seated Spinal Twist:

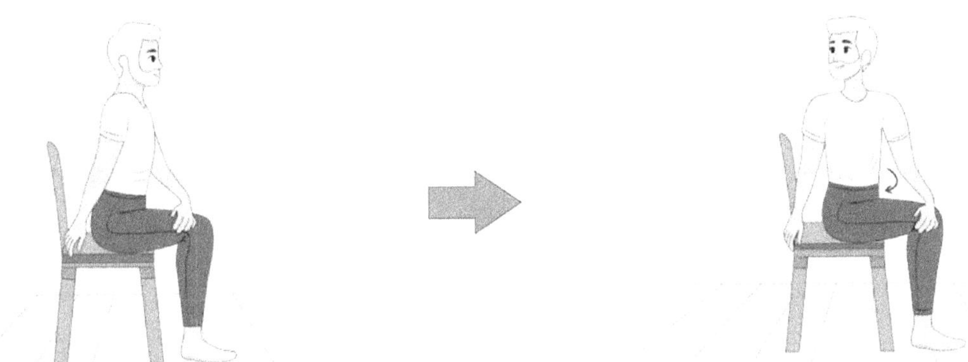

1. Sit firmly with feet flat. Place your right hand on the left knee and the left hand behind you for support.

● Inhale to lengthen the spine further before beginning the twist.

2. Exhale and gently twist to the left, using your hands as leverage to deepen the twist without forcing.

● Look over your left shoulder to enhance the spinal twist.

Repetition: Hold five deep breaths, focusing on the stretch and maintaining a tall spine, then switch sides

Caution: Twist should be gentle and controlled, originating from the base of the spine.

3) Chair Pigeon Pose:

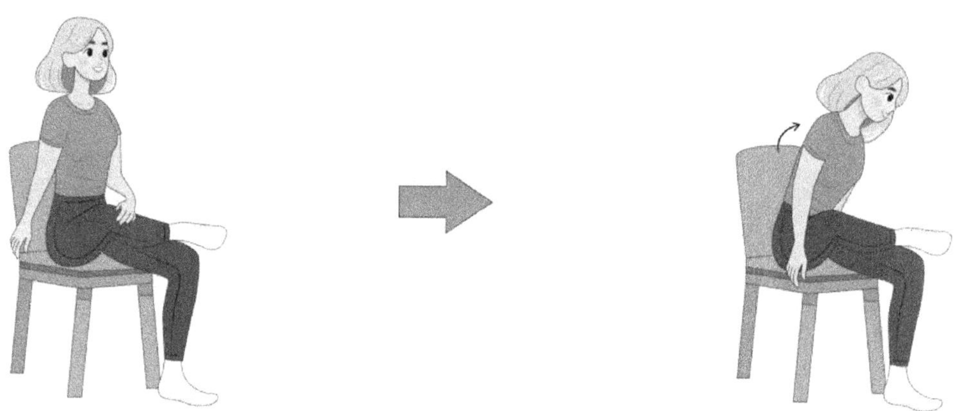

1. Sit with legs uncrossed, maintaining a straight spine.

2. Gently lift your right ankle, placing it on your left knee and allowing the right knee to open to the side.

- Flex your foot to ensure protection for the knee.

3. Inhale to prepare, then exhale as you lean forward slightly, hinging at the hips to deepen your right hip and glute stretch.

- Keep your back flat, imagining a string pulling you forward from your chest.

Repetition: Hold for five breaths before switching sides, using the breath to ease into the stretch.

Caution: Maintain a gentle stretch to avoid knee or hip strain.

After Exercises: Engage in visualization and meditation, then Coordination of Intentional Movements.

Day 10: Integration of Strength and Flexibility Poses

Goal: Balance strength and flexibility

Before Exercises: As in Day 8

DAY 10

EXERCISE	SETS
☐ Tree Pose	5 brs/side
☐ Sun Salutations	x3–5
☐ Warrior II	5 brs/side

1) Seated Tree Pose:

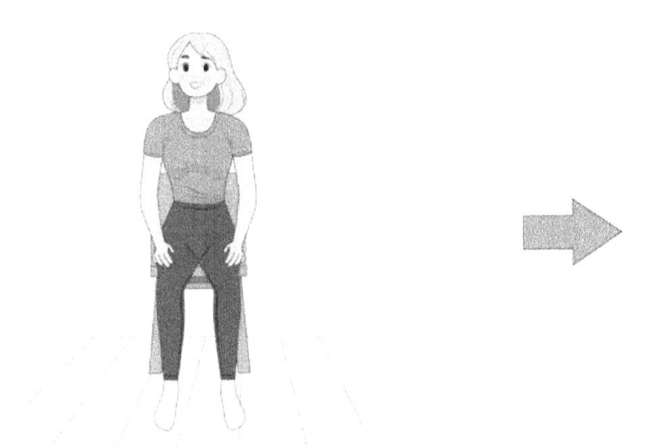

1. Sit with both feet flat on the floor

2. Gently place your right foot on your left thigh, just above the knee, opening your right knee to the side.

● Ensure your spine remains straight, promoting an upright posture.

3. Press your palms together at the heart center, maintaining an upright posture.

4. Focus on your balance and breathe deeply, holding the pose for five breaths.

5. Carefully lower your leg and switch sides, repeating the pose with the left foot on the right thigh.

Repetition: Hold for five breaths on each side.

Caution: Ensure your foot is placed on the thigh, not the knee, to avoid pressure on the knee joint.

2) Chair Sun Salutations:

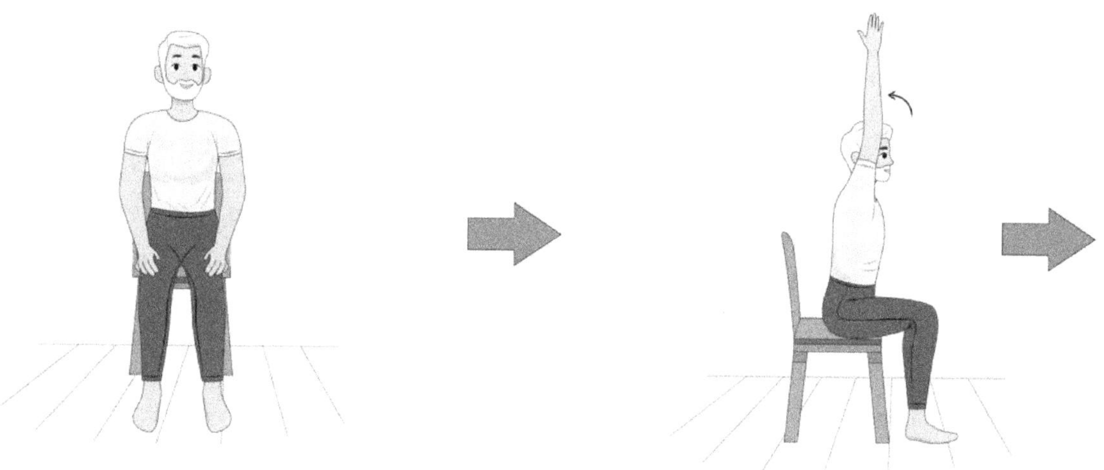

1. Seated Mountain Pose: Begin with a deep breath, sitting tall and grounded.

2. Seated Upward Salute: Inhale, lifting your arms to the sides and above your head, joining your hands if comfortable.

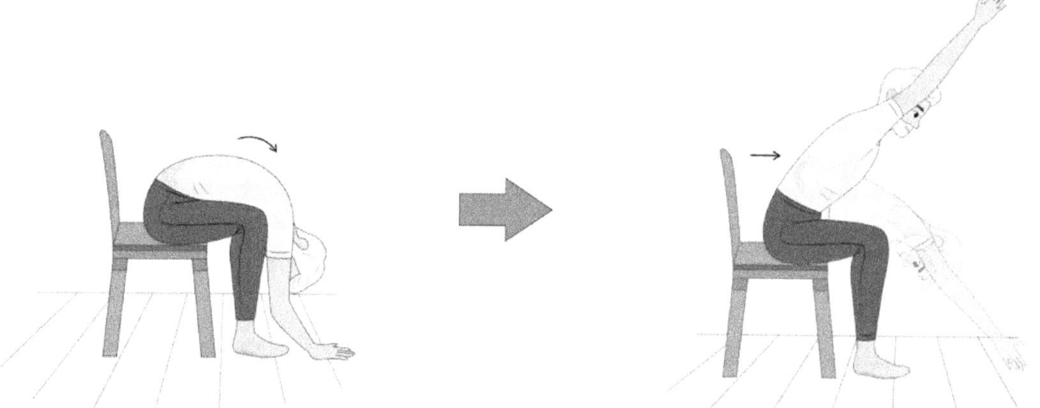

3. Seated Forward Fold: Exhale, hinging at the hips to lean forward, reaching toward your legs. Let your head hang naturally.

● Place your hands wherever they can rest without strain, ensuring comfort.

4. Seated Half Lift: Inhale, lifting your torso halfway up, hands above your head, or on your knees if you feel tension, straightening your back.

5. Return to Seated Forward Fold: Exhale and fold again, releasing tension.

Repetition: Flow through this sequence 3-5 times

Caution: Move within your comfort range to avoid overstretching or straining, especially in your neck and back.

3) Chair Warrior II:

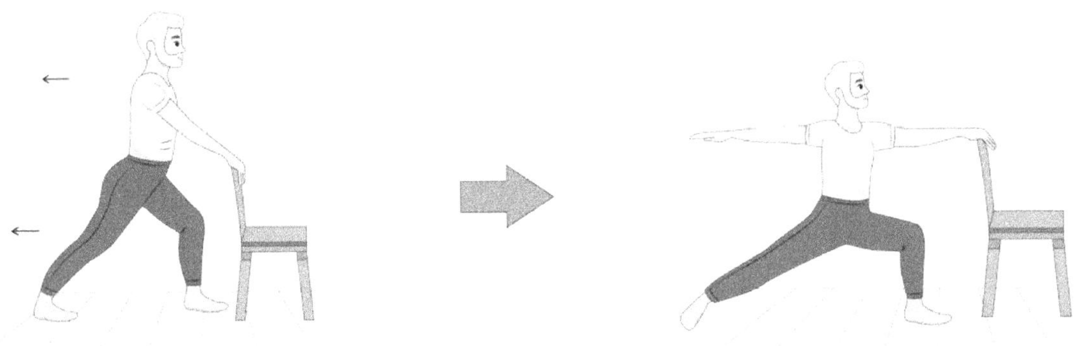

1. Stand beside a chair for needed support.

2. Extend your right leg back, keeping your left foot forward and both feet flat.

- Keep your front knee aligned directly over your ankle.

3. Bend your left knee, ensuring it's directly above the ankle, while your right leg remains straight.

4. Extend your arms to the sides, parallel to the floor, and turn your head to gaze over your left hand.

Repetition: Hold the pose for five deep breaths, feeling the stretch and maintaining balance. Return to the starting position and switch sides, extending the left leg back and bending the right knee.

Caution:

- Keep the bent knee from extending past the toes to avoid strain.
- Use the chair for support to maintain balance if necessary.

After Exercises: Continue as in Day 8.

<u>Day 11: Seated and Standing Poses Combination</u>

Goal: Enhance coordination and strength

Before Exercises: As in previous days.

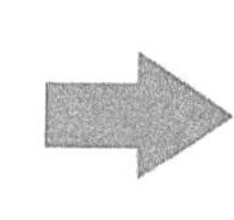

1) Standing Triangle Pose

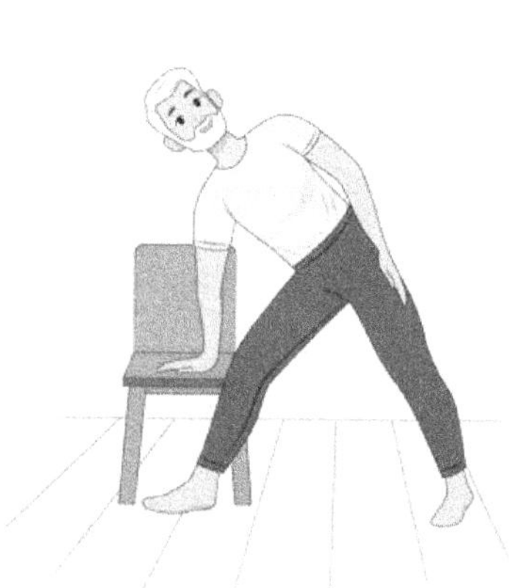 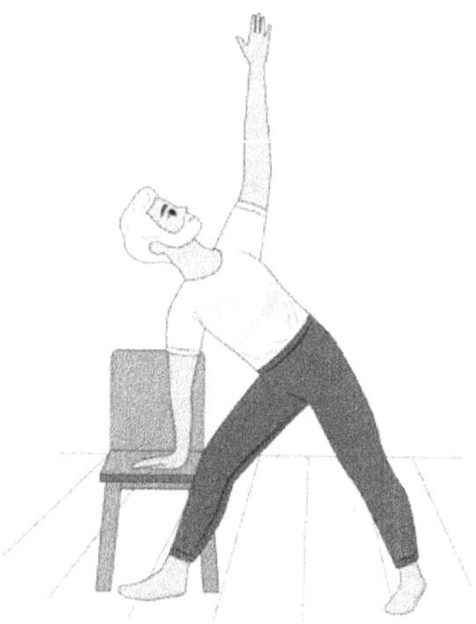

1. Stand beside a chair, using it for stability.
- Place the chair on your side to ensure it is easily accessible

2. Lean towards the chair, placing your other hand on it for support.

3. Ensure a gentle lean without putting all your weight on the chair.

4. Lift one arm over your head to stretch the side of your body, reaching upwards.
- Keep your feet firmly on the ground to maintain balance.

5. Hold this position for five deep breaths, focusing on the stretch.

Repetition: After five breaths, stand and switch arms to repeat on the opposite side.

Caution:
- Use the chair only for light support to prevent any strain.
- Keep your movements smooth and controlled to avoid jerky motions that could lead to injury.

2) Seated Eagle Pose:

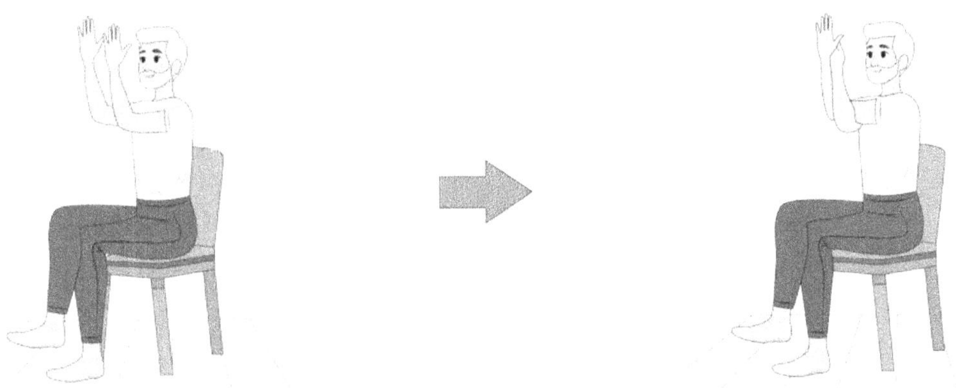

1. Sit upright in the chair, cross your right thigh over your left thigh as much as possible.

2. Bring your left arm underneath your right arm, then bend your elbows to press your palms together or as closely as possible.

- Focus on maintaining balance and alignment in the pose, keeping your spine straight.

3. Hold this position for 30 seconds, breathing deeply and focusing on the stretch in your shoulders and hips.

- Carefully switch sides, repeating the pose with the left thigh over the right and the right arm under the left.

Repetition: Hold for 30 seconds on each side.

Caution:
- Ensure your spine remains straight to avoid slouching.
- Modify the leg and arm positions if you experience any discomfort.

3) Standing Chair Pose:

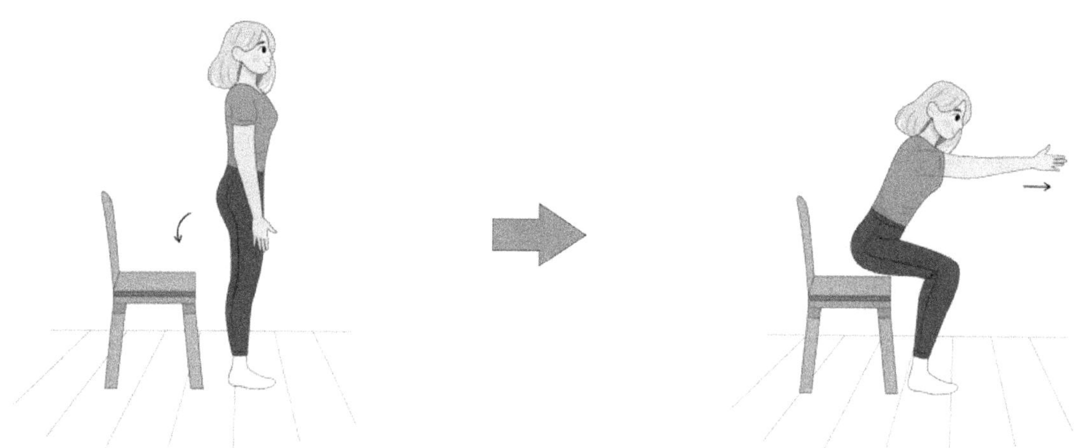

1. Stand in front of a chair as if you're about to sit down, but stop just before your seat touches the chair.

● Make sure your feet are shoulder-width apart for stability.

2. Extend your arms at shoulder height, keeping them parallel to the ground.

● Engage your core by drawing your belly button towards your spine to support your lower back.

3. Bend your knees slightly, as if hovering above the chair, and hold this position for five deep breaths.

● Focus on keeping your thighs engaged and your weight evenly distributed across your feet.

Repetition: After holding five breaths, slowly straighten your legs to return to standing.

Caution:

● Ensure the chair is stable and won't move during the exercise.

● If you feel any strain in your knees, adjust the depth of your squat.

● Inhale as you prepare to stand, using your leg strength to lift yourself.

After Exercises: As in previous days.

Day 12: Focused Breathing with Movement

Goal: Synchronize breath with movements.

Before Exercises: As in previous days.

DAY 12

	EXERCISE	SETS
☐	Cat-Cow	x5 cycles
☐	Breath of Joy	x5 cycles
☐	Brs. Awareness	5 minutes

1) Seated Cat-Cow with Breath:

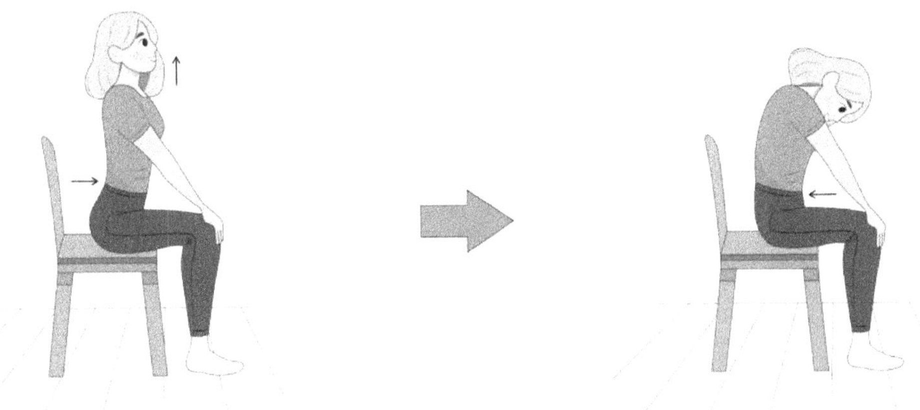

1. Inhale deeply, arching your back and tilting your head and tailbone towards the ceiling (Cow position).

- Ensure a smooth transition into the arch.

2. Exhale fully, rounding your spine, drawing your chin to your chest, and tucking your tailbone under (Cat position).

- Match the rounding of the back with a complete exhalation.

Repetition: Repeat this fluid motion for five cycles, focusing on syncing each movement with your breath.

Caution:
- Move gently to prevent straining the back.
- Make sure to synchronize your breath and movement for the most significant benefit

2) Breath of Joy:

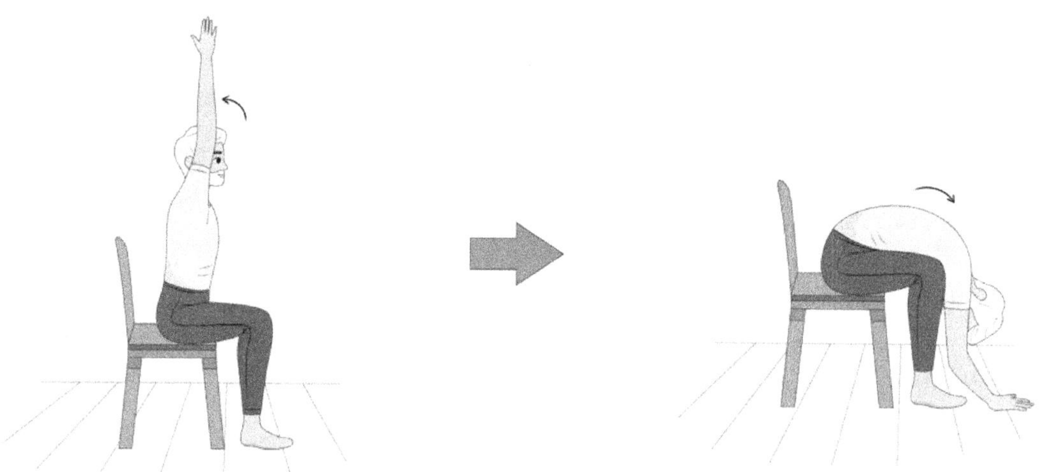

1. Sit on the chair with feet shoulder-width apart. Inhale in three short parts, lifting your arms in front, to the sides, and then above your head.

2. On a complete exhale, bend forward from the hips, bringing your arms down and back.
- Inhale in three parts should be smooth and energizing.

Repetition: Repeat this dynamic movement for five cycles, allowing the breath to guide the energy and flow.

Caution:
- Bend from the hips to avoid strain on the back.
- If dizzy, pause and resume normal breathing.

3) Seated Breath Awareness:

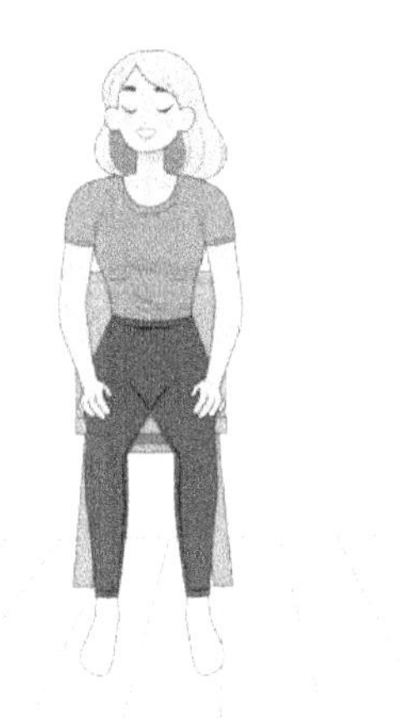

1. Focus on your natural breath, observing its flow in and out without trying to change it.

2. Notice the rise and fall of your abdomen with each breath to enhance mindfulness.

3. Continue this focused awareness for five minutes, returning your attention to your breath whenever it wanders.

- If your mind wanders, gently guide it back to your breath without judgment.

Repetition: Five minutes.

Caution:

- Ensure you're in a comfortable position to avoid unnecessary strain during the practice.
- Maintain a gentle focus, avoiding over-concentration.

After Exercises: As in previous days.

Day 13: Advanced Seated Twists and Side Bends

Goal: Deepen spinal stretches

Before Exercises: As in previous days.

DAY 13

EXERCISE	SETS
☐ Marichyasana	5 brs/side
☐ Side Stretch	5 brs/side
☐ Revolved Pose	5 brs/side

1) Seated Marichyasana:

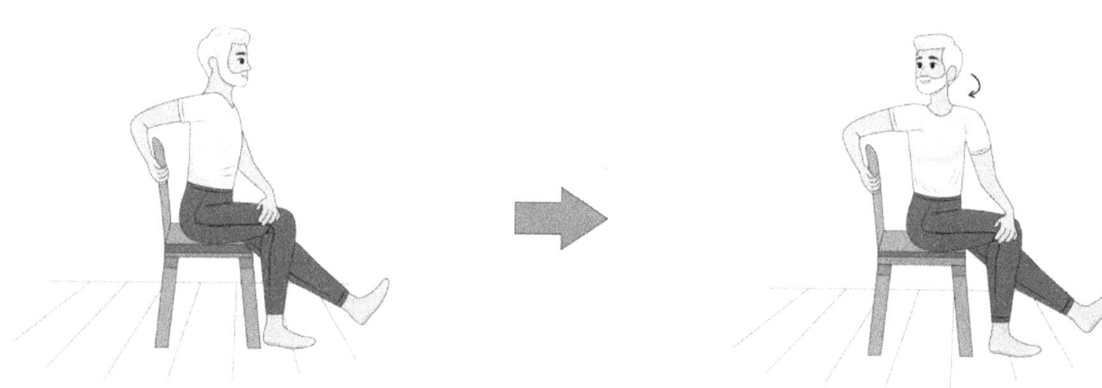

1. Sit with both legs extended in front of you.

2. Bend your right knee, placing the right foot flat on the floor, close to your body.

3. Twist your torso to the right, bringing your left arm over the right knee.

● Use the arm to gently deepen the twist to keep both sit bones on the chair seat.

Repetition: Hold the pose for five breaths, focusing on the twist and stretch in your back. Slowly release and switch sides, repeating the twist with the left knee bent.

Caution:

● Avoid straining your back or neck;

● the twist should be gentle and comfortable.

2) Seated Side Stretch with Arms Overhead:

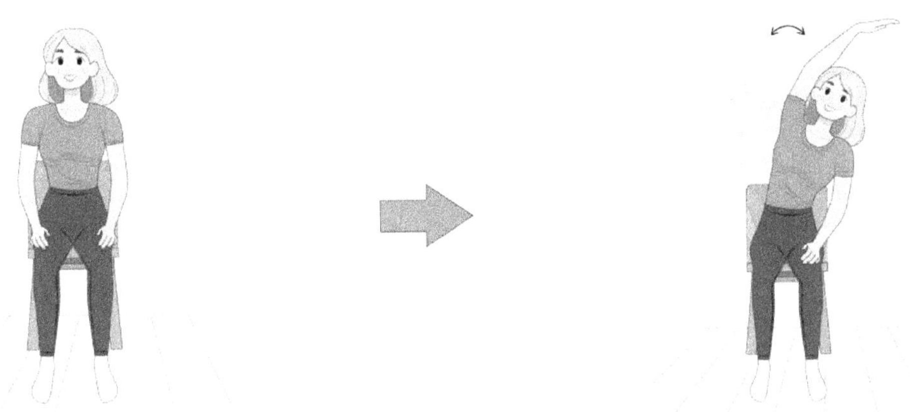

1. Sit upright and extend your right arm overhead, bending your torso to the left side.

● Keep your left hand on the chair for balance, if needed.

2. Focus on stretching the right side of your torso, keeping both sit bones grounded.

Repetition: Hold for five breaths on each side

Caution: Ensure smooth movement and avoid collapsing into the lower side.

3) Revolved Chair Pose:

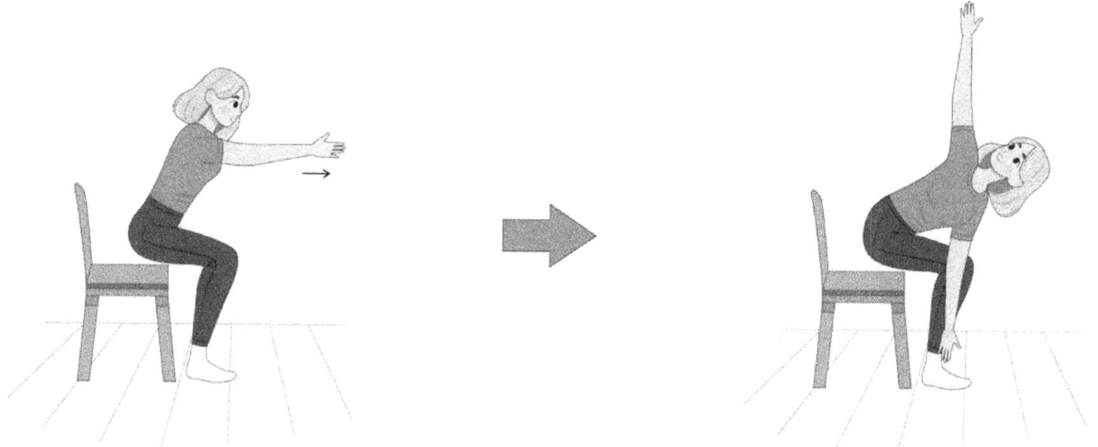

1. Lower your hips as if sitting back in a chair, keeping your weight in your heels.

2. Twist your torso to the right, extending your left arm forward and your right arm back, aligning them with your shoulders.

● Keep your spine long and core engaged to support the twist.

3. Stretch your top arm (right arm) upwards while the other hand (left hand) reaches down as if touching the floor, enhancing the twist.

Repetition: Hold this pose for five deep breaths on each side, maintaining the bend in your knees and the twist in your torso.

Caution:

● Keep knees aligned with toes to avoid knee strain.

● Maintain a solid core to support the spine during the twist.

After Exercises: As in previous days.

<u>**Day 14: Review of Week's Poses and Techniques**</u>

Goal: Consolidate learning from the week.

Before Exercises: As in previous days.

Routine: Practice a selected combination of poses from the week. Focus on integrating strength, flexibility, and breathwork learned during the week.

DAY 14

EXERCISE	SETS
☐ Selected	as in
☐ Combination of	previous
☐ Poses the week	times

Week 3: Balance and Coordination

Reflecting on Week 2's journey, where we focused on building flexibility and strength, we now transition to Week 3, emphasizing balance and coordination. This new week aims to progressively enhance these essential skills, which are fundamental in our daily movements and integral to yoga practice. As we delve into exercises that challenge and refine our balance, particularly in standing poses with chair support, we'll continue to monitor our progress, assessing how our bodies adapt and respond. Week 3 is vital in our chair yoga journey, contributing to our overall coordination and physical confidence.

Week 3 Planner

Day	Routine	Goal	Time Spent	Notes
Day 15	Balance Exercises in Seated Position	Improve balance while seated		
Day 16	Coordination Drills with Arm and Leg Movements	Enhance limb coordination		
Day 17	Standing Poses Using Chair for Support	Practice balance in standing poses		
Day 18	Eye Coordination and Focused Movements	Develop eye-hand coordination		
Day 19	Combining Balance and Breathing Techniques	Integrate breath with balance		
Day 20	Dynamic Movement Flow for Coordination	Improve overall body coordination		

Day	Routine	Goal	Time Spent	Notes
Day 21	Rest Day with Gentle Stretching	Allow the body to recover and reflect		

<u>Day 15: Balance Exercises in Seated Position</u>

Goal: Improve balance while seated

Before Exercises: Begin with Seated Mindful Foundation and breathing exercises, then warm-up movements for 3-5 minutes.

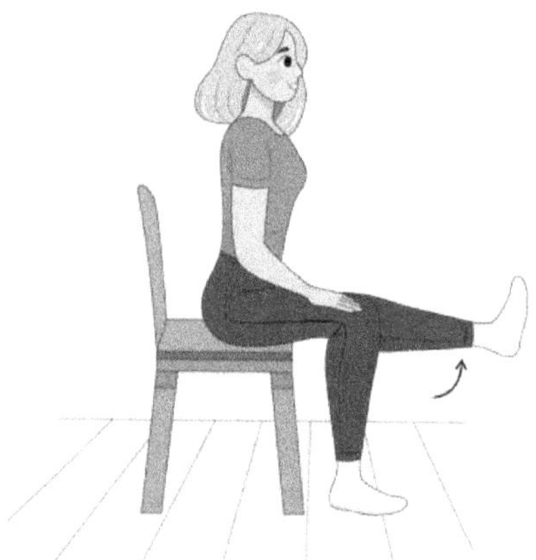

1. Seated Single-Leg Extensions:

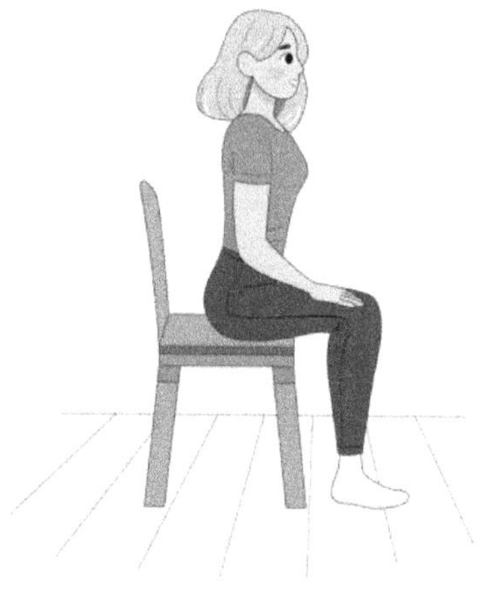 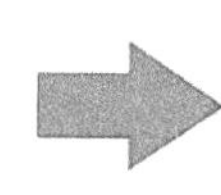

1. Extend one leg straight before you, aiming to keep it parallel to the floor.

- Engage your thigh muscles to maintain the extension.

2. Hold the position for three breaths, focusing on balance and the engagement of your leg muscles.

3. Lower the leg gently and switch to the other leg, repeating the extension.

Repetition: Hold each leg for three breaths.

Caution: Ensure you maintain an upright posture to avoid straining your back.

2) Seated Side Leg Raises:

1. Lift one leg to the side, keeping the rest of your body as still and straight as possible.

- The lift doesn't have to be high; focus on the quality of the movement.

2. Hold for three breaths, engaging the muscles on the side of your hip.

3. Lower the leg and switch to the other, repeating the raise.

Repetition: Hold each leg for three breaths.

Caution: Keep your torso straight and avoid leaning to the opposite side to maintain balance.

3). Seated Torso Twists:

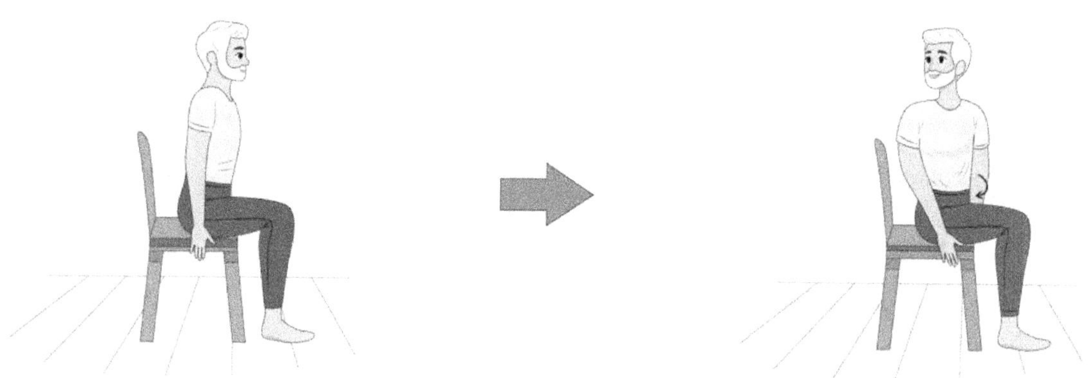

1. Sit with both feet flat on the floor, spine straight.

2. Place your hands on the edges of the chair for support as you twist your torso to one side.

● Use the chair for leverage to deepen the twist gently.

3. Hold the twist for three breaths, focusing on the stretch through your spine.

4. Return to the center and repeat the twist on the opposite side.

Repetition: Hold the twist for three breaths on each side.

Caution: Twist from the base of your spine, moving upwards; avoid straining your neck.

After Exercises: Engage in visualization and meditation, then Coordination of Intentional Movements.

Day 16: Coordination Drills with Arm and Leg Movements

DAY 16

EXERCISE	SETS
☐ Arm & leg raise	3 brs/side
☐ Marching	1 minute
☐ Cross Body	3 brs/side

Goal: Enhance limb coordination

Before Exercises: As in previous days.

1) Opposite Arm and Leg Raises:

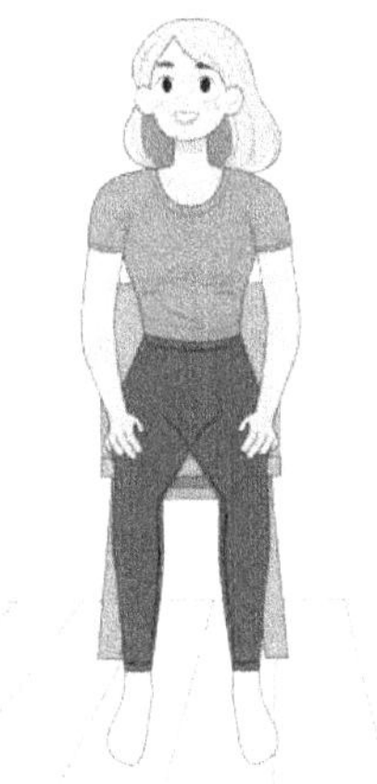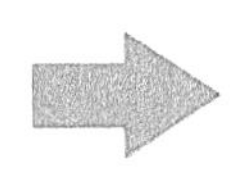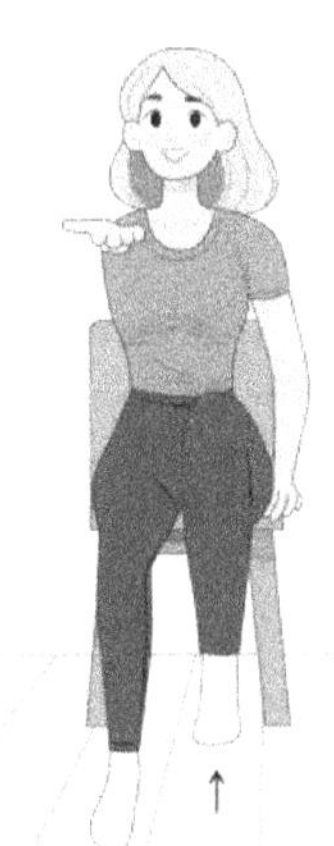

1. Sit upright on a chair.

2. Lift your right arm and left leg simultaneously, aiming for a balanced and smooth lift.

● Focus on engaging your core for stability.

3. Lower them gently and then lift your left arm and right leg, maintaining smooth, controlled movements.

Repetition: Continue alternating sides, performing the movement for three breaths on each side.

Caution: Control your movements to maintain balance and prevent any strain.

2) Seated Marching with Arm Swings:

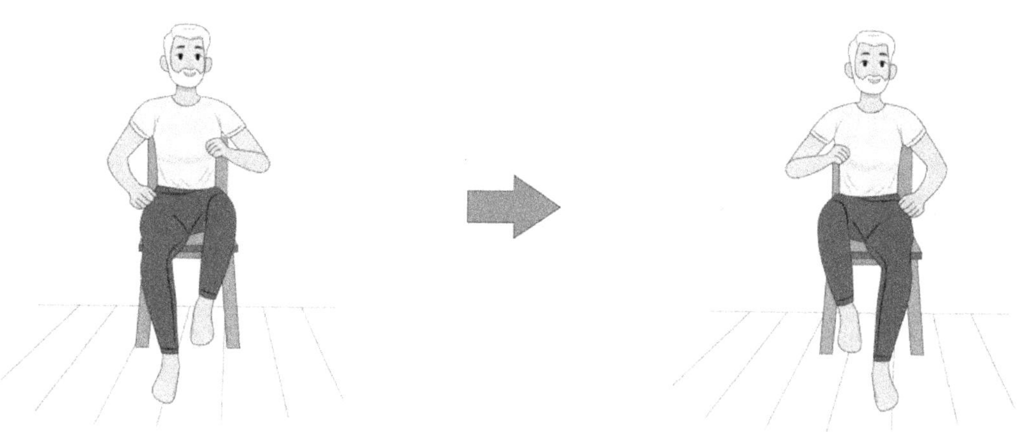

1. Begin by simulating a marching motion, lifting your knees alternately as if marching on the spot.

● Add opposite arm swings to mimic natural walking or marching movements.

2. Continue this coordinated motion for a minute, focusing on the rhythm and coordination between your arms and legs.

Repetition: Continue for one minute.

Caution: Keep your posture upright to engage the core and support your back.

3) Cross-Body Reaches:

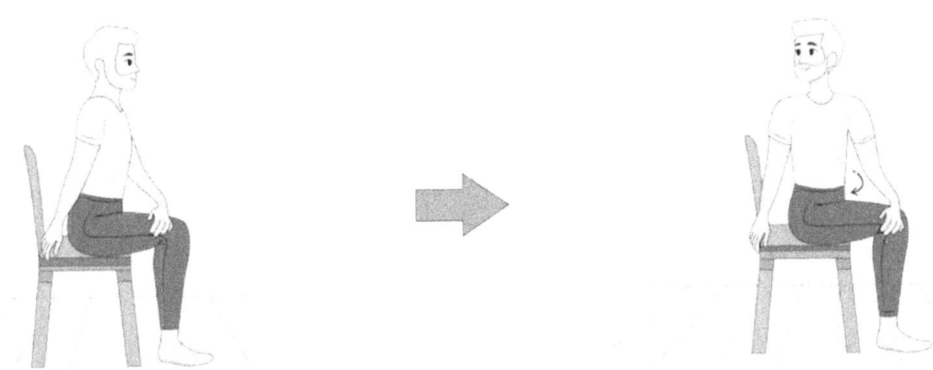

1. Sit firmly with feet flat. Place your right hand on the left knee and the left hand behind you for support.

● Inhale to lengthen the spine further before beginning the twist.

2. Exhale and gently twist to the left, using your hands as leverage to deepen the twist without forcing.

● Look over your left shoulder to enhance the spinal twist.

Repetition: Three breaths on each side alternation.

Caution: Move within a comfortable range of motion to avoid overstretching.

After Exercises: As in Day 15.

<u>Day 17: Standing Poses Using Chair for Support</u>

Goal: Practice balance in standing poses

Before Exercises: Follow the same routine as Day 15

1) Chair-Supported Tree Pose:

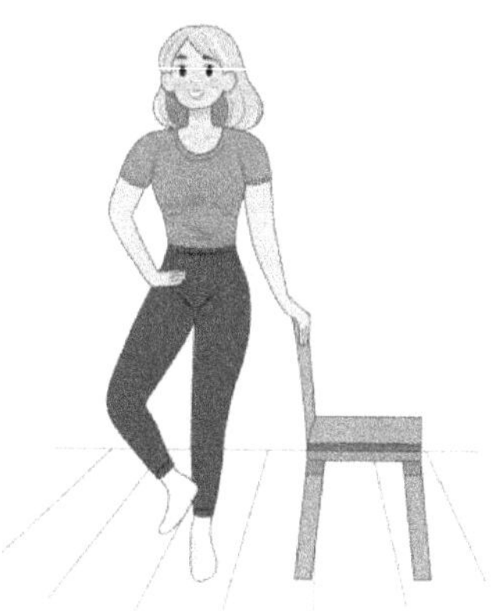 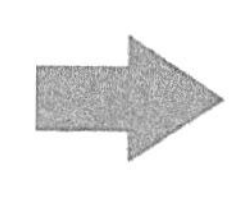 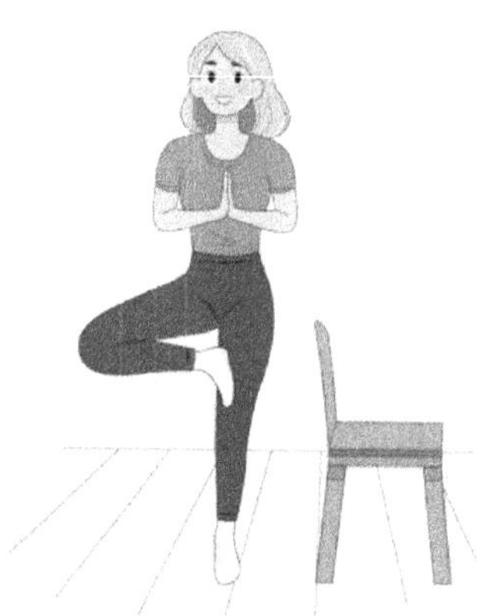

1. Stand beside a chair for balance. Place your weight on your right leg, firmly planting your foot on the ground.

● Place your left foot on your right thigh, avoiding the knee area to protect the joint.

2. With your suitable leg stable, bring your palms together in front of your chest in prayer, maintaining balance and focusing on your breath.

● If balancing is challenging, use the chair for support with one hand.

Repetition: Hold for five breaths on each side

Caution: Use the chair for stability to prevent falls.

2) Chair-Assisted Warrior III:

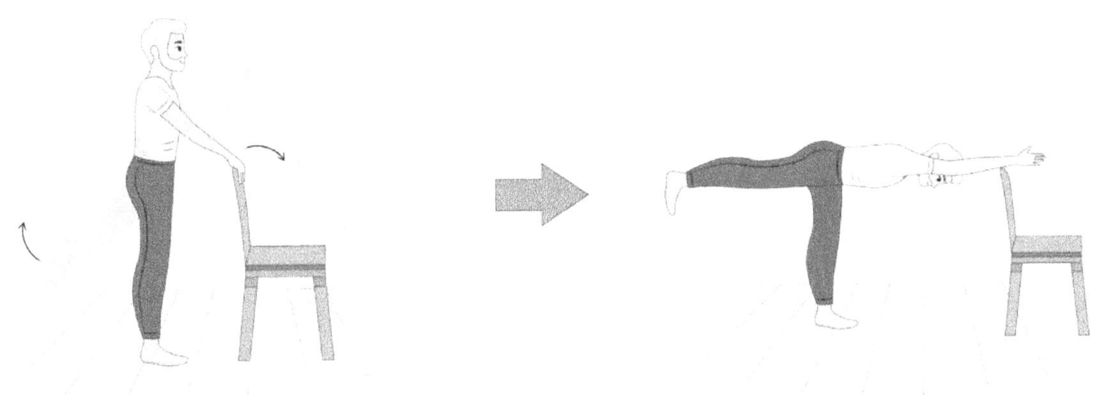

1. Stand facing the chair, using it for support

2. Lean forward, placing your hands on the chair.

3. Extend your right leg back, aiming to form a T-shape with your body, keeping the hip of the lifted leg facing down.

4. Hold for five breaths, focusing on the stretch and balance.

Repetition: Hold for five breaths on each side.

Caution: Keep the supporting leg slightly bent to avoid locking the knee.

3) Standing Leg Lifts:

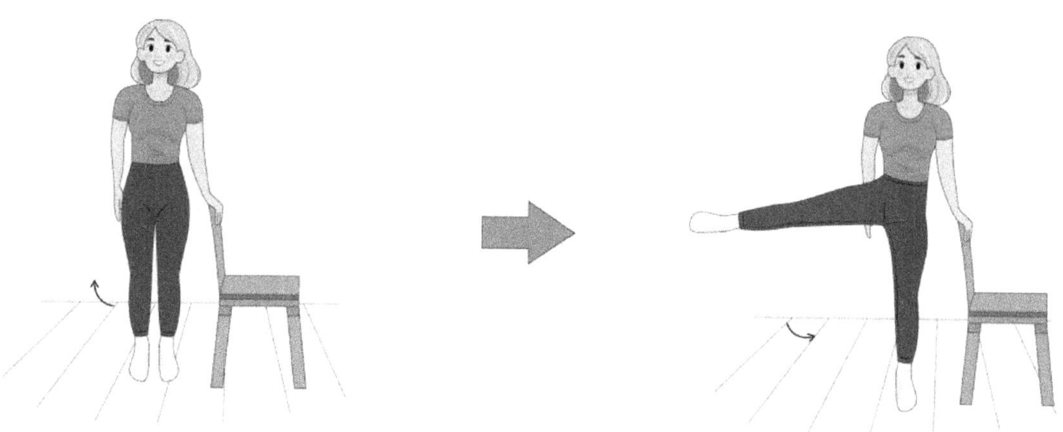

1. Stand behind the chair, holding the back for support.

2. Lift your right leg to the side, keeping it straight, then swing it back slightly.

● Focus on smooth movements and maintaining balance.

Repetition: Perform five lifts on each side.

Caution: Move within a comfortable range to avoid straining the muscles

After Exercises: As in Day 15

Day 18: Eye Coordination and Focused Movements

DAY 18

EXERCISE	SETS
☐ Eye Tracking	3-5 minute
☐ Turn Eye Focus	3-5 minute
☐ Coordination	3-5 minute

Goal: Develop eye-hand coordination

Before Exercises: As in previous days.

1) Seated Eye Tracking:

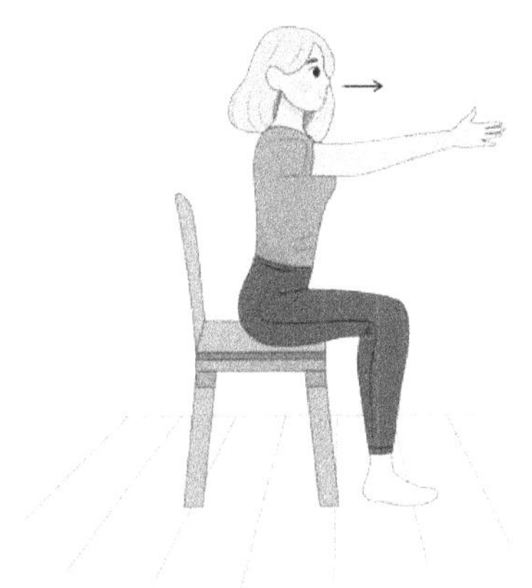

1. Sit comfortably and hold your thumb about an arm's length from your face.

2. Slowly move your thumb from side to side, keeping your head still.

3. Follow the movement with your eyes, focusing on your thumb throughout

Repetition: Continue for 3-5 minutes.

Caution: Ensure smooth movements to avoid straining your eyes.

2) Head Turns with Eye Focus:

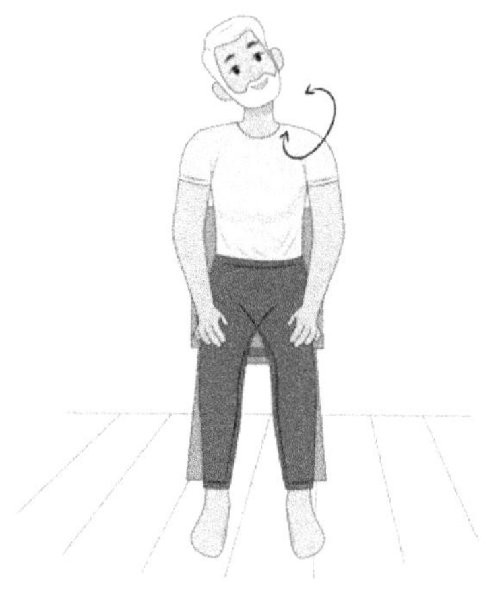

1. Choose a distant project as your focal point.

2. Turn your head slowly from side to side, trying to focus on the object each time your head turns.

3. Coordinate the head movements with your eye focus, maintaining a steady gaze.

Repetition: Practice for 3-5 minute.

Caution: Move your head gently to avoid neck strain.

3) Hand-Eye Coordination Drill:

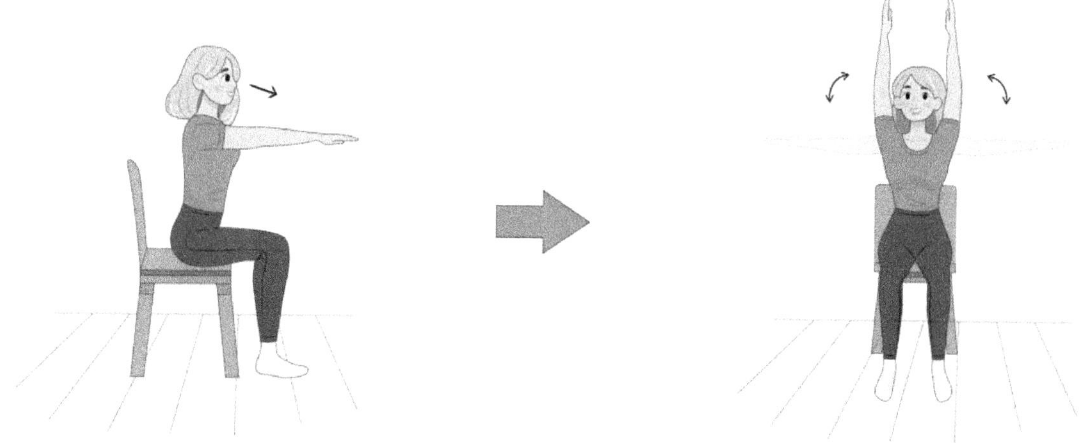

1. Extend your arms before you, then move them in different directions (up, down, side to side).

2. Keep your head still, following the movements with your eyes.

3. Focus on the coordination between your eye movements and hand movements.

Repetition: Continue for 3-5 minutes.

Caution: Control your movements carefully to maintain focus and prevent fatigue.

Day 19: Combining Balance and Breathing Techniques

Goal: Integrate breath with balance

Before Exercises: As in previous days.

DAY 19

EXERCISE	SETS
☐ Balancing in leg	5 brs/leg
☐ Flow with Sync	5 minutes
☐ Nostril Breathing	5 minutes

1) Balanced Breathing on One Leg:

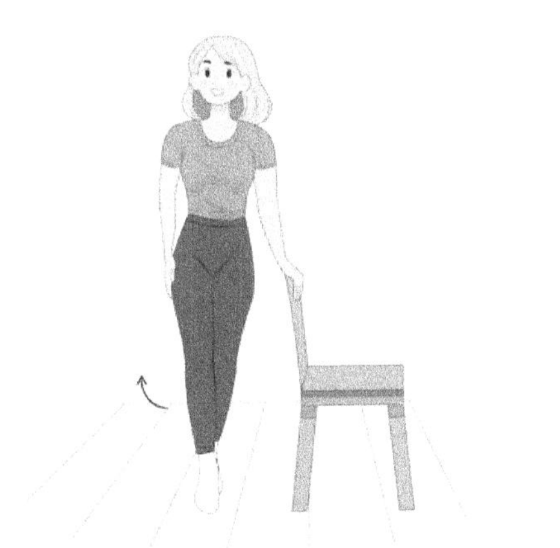
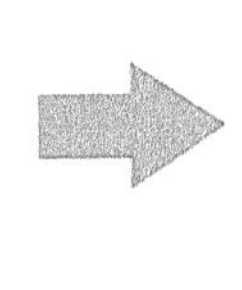
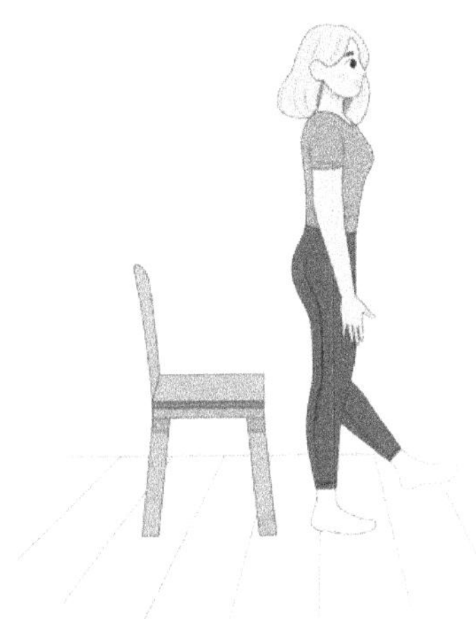

1. Stand firmly on your right leg, gently raising your left foot. Find a point ahead of you to maintain focus and balance.

● Keep your supporting leg slightly bent to avoid locking the knee.

2. Begin to breathe deeply and steadily, focusing on maintaining calm and even living as you balance.

3. After holding for five breaths, carefully switch to your left leg and repeat the process, aiming for the same focus and balance.

Repetition: Hold for five breaths on each leg.

Caution:
● Use a chair or wall for support if needed.
● Ensure your lifted foot doesn't rest against the knee of your standing leg.

2) Chair Yoga Flow with Breath Sync:

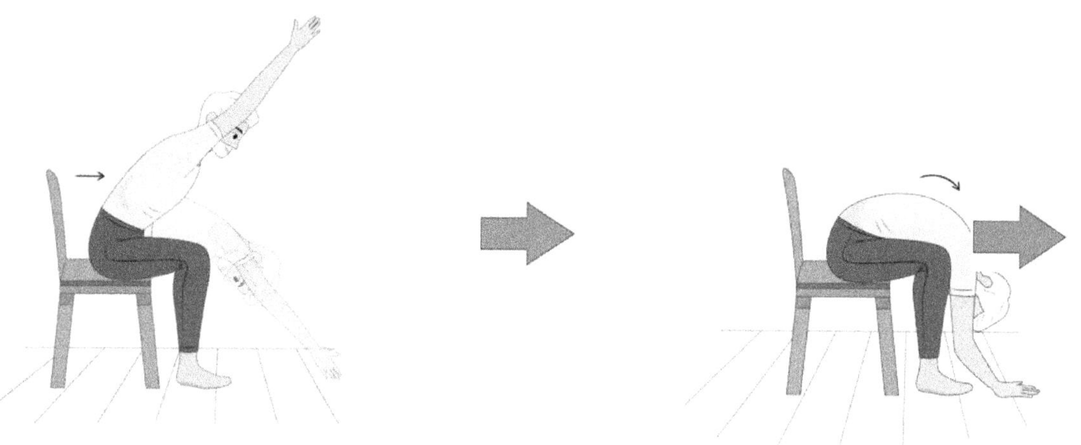

1.   Sit in a chair with your back straight and feet firmly on the ground.

2.   Inhale Deeply: Sit tall, expanding your chest and filling your lungs with air. Keep your spine aligned and arms above your head.

3. Forward Bend Transition: Exhale slowly, hinging at the hips to lean forward gently, stretching your back.

● Let your arms hang loosely towards the floor to enhance the stretch.

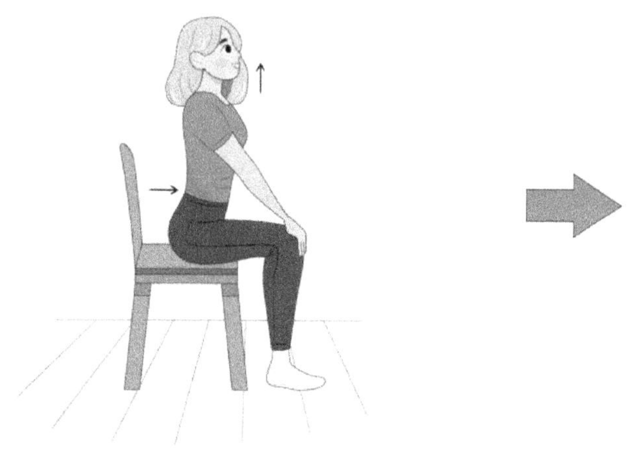

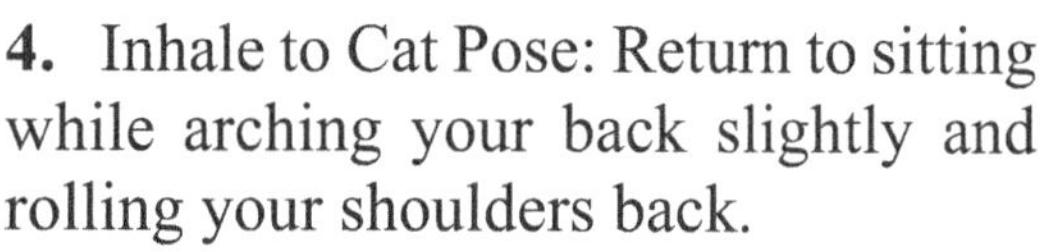

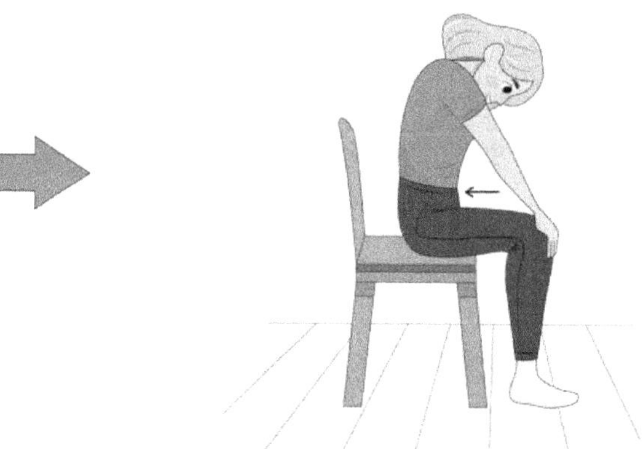

4. Inhale to Cat Pose: Return to sitting while arching your back slightly and rolling your shoulders back.

5. Exhale to Cow Pose: Round your spine, tucking your chin to your chest, emphasizing the curve in your back.

● Ensure smooth transitions between Cat and Cow, mirroring the rhythm of your breath.

Repetition: Flow through the movements for 5 minutes, using your breath to guide each transition.

Caution:

● Move within a comfortable range, avoiding any strain.

● Maintain a grounded posture to ensure stability and support.

3) Seated Alternate Nostril Breathing:

1. Sit comfortably with your spine erect and shoulders relaxed. Use your right thumb to close your right nostril gently.

2. Inhale deeply through your left nostril, then use your fingers to close it, opening your right nostril to exhale slowly.

3. Inhale through the right nostril, then close it and exhale through the left to complete one cycle.

Repetition: Continue this breathing pattern for 5 minutes, focusing on the flow and balance of your breath.

Caution:

- Ensure gentle pressure on the nostrils to avoid discomfort.
- If you feel dizzy or uncomfortable, pause and breathe normally.

After Exercises: As in previous days.

<u>Day 20: Dynamic Movement Flow for Coordination</u>

Goal: Improve overall body coordination

Before Exercises: As in previous days.

DAY 20

	EXERCISE	SETS
☐	Seat to Stand	x10
☐	Flowing Sun	3-5 minute
☐	Walk in Place	3-5 minute

1) Seated to Standing Transitions

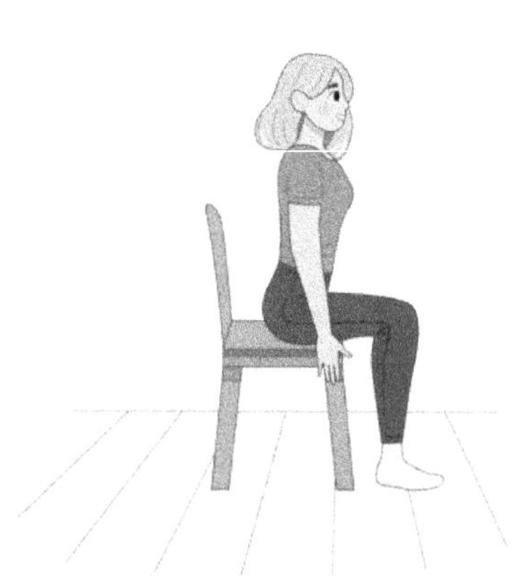  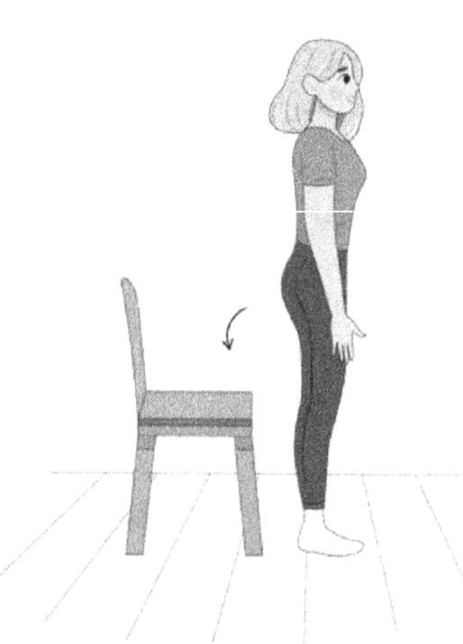

1. Begin seated with your feet firmly planted on the floor, hip-width apart. Engage your core muscles to prepare for the lift.

• Push through your heels to stand, using your leg muscles rather than leveraging with your arms.

2. Slowly rise to a standing position, focusing on maintaining a straight spine and balanced posture.

3. Gently lower yourself back to the seated position, controlling the descent to engage your muscles fully.

• Ensure the chair is directly behind you to avoid missing it as you sit.

Repetition: Smoothly perform this transition ten times.

Caution:

• Ensure your chair is stable and won't slide.

• Move slowly to maintain balance and prevent any sudden movements.

2) Flowing Chair Sun Salutations:

1. Start in a seated mountain pose, arms lifting and taking a deep breath. As you exhale, transition into a seated forward bend, reaching toward your toes.

2. Forward Bend Transition: Exhale slowly, hinging at the hips to lean forward gently, stretching your back.

● Inhale, lifting your torso and extending your arms for a slight backbend.

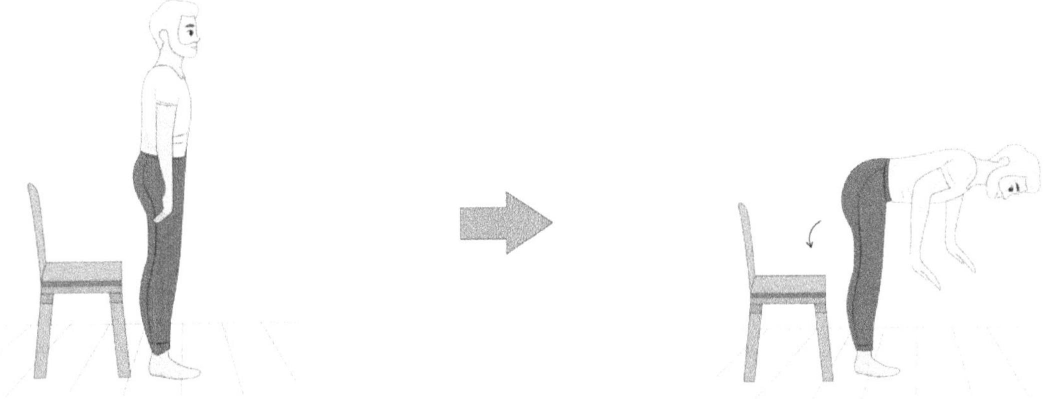

3. Stand up, flowing into a standing mountain pose, then into a standing forward bend on your next exhale.

4. Gradually return to standing, transitioning back into the seated poses, syncing each movement with your breath.

Repetition: Flow through the sequence for 3-5 minutes.

Caution:

● Adapt poses as needed to fit your flexibility and comfort level

● Ensure movements are fluid to avoid strain.

3) Balanced Walking in Place:

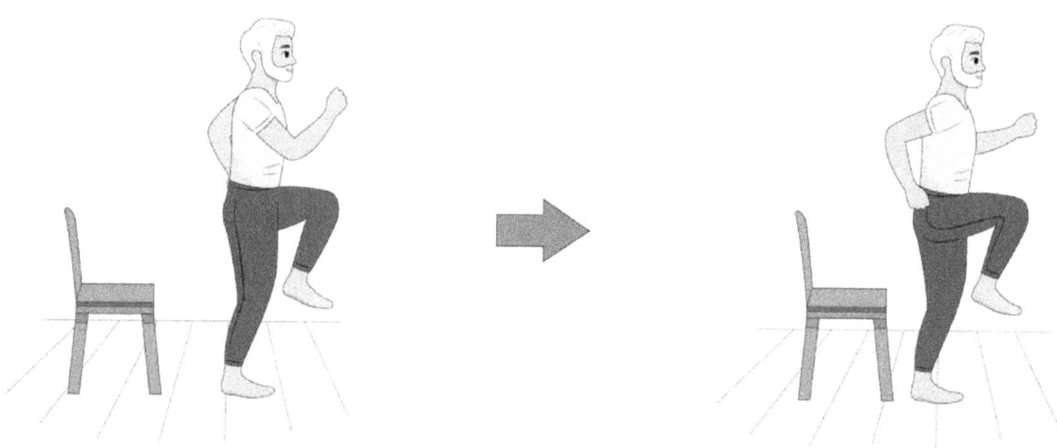

1. Stand with feet hip-width apart, engaging your core for stability. Begin to lift your knees high, mimicking a marching motion.

● Add arm swings, coordinating the opposite arm to the leg to simulate natural walking motion.

2. Focus on lifting your knees comfortably and maintaining an upright posture throughout the exercise.

3. Continue this walking in place, ensuring each step is controlled and balanced for 5 minutes.

● Pay attention to your foot placement, providing a soft landing each time.

Repetition: Continue for 5 minutes, maintaining rhythm and balance.

Caution:

● Keep your space clear of any obstacles.
● If you feel any discomfort, reduce the height of your knee lifts.

After Exercises: As in previous days.

Day 21: Rest Day with Gentle Stretching

Goal: Allow the body to recover and reflect

Before Exercises: As in previous days.

DAY 21

EXERCISE	SETS
☐ Forward Bend	5 breaths
☐ Side Stretch	5 brs/side
☐ Meditation	5 minutes

1) Seated Forward Bend:

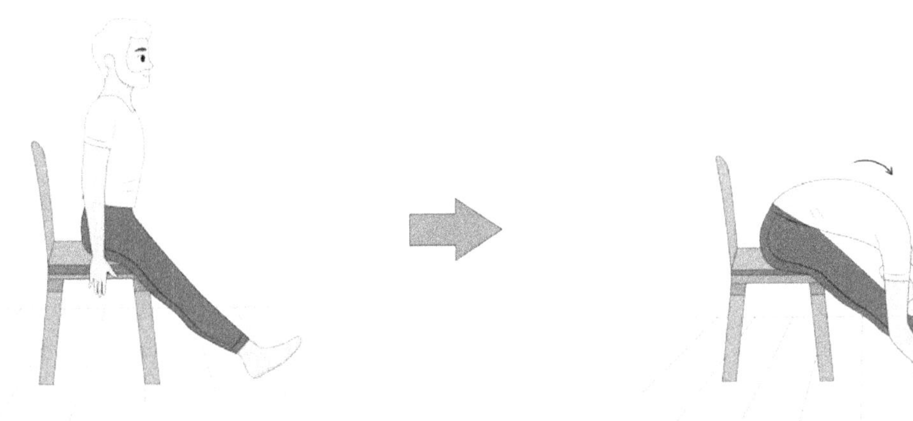

1. Sit with your legs straight out in front.

2. Breathe in and raise your arms to lengthen your spine before bending.

3. Breathe out, bend your hips towards your toes, keeping your back straight.

● Aim for hip movement rather than back rounding to reach further.

4. Stretch towards your toes as far as feels, aiming for a stretch in your hamstrings and back.

Repetition: Hold the forward lean for five deep breaths, allowing each exhale to relax you further into the stretch

Caution: Avoid rounding the back too much; aim for a hinged motion from the hips.

2) Seated Side Stretches:

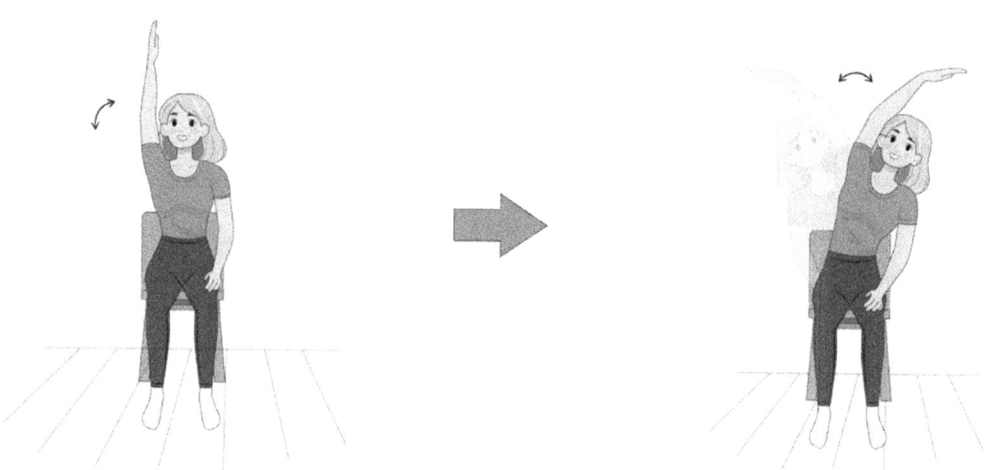

1. Sit upright and raise your right arm overhead. Inhale deeply.

2. As you exhale, gently lean to the left, stretching the right side of your torso. Keep your left hand on the chair seat for support.

● Ensure both sit bones remain in contact with the seat to maintain balance.

Repetition: Hold the stretch for five deep breaths, then switch sides, stretching the left side of your torso.

Caution: Do not overextend; the goal is a gentle stretch along the side of your body.

3) Guided Relaxation or Meditation:

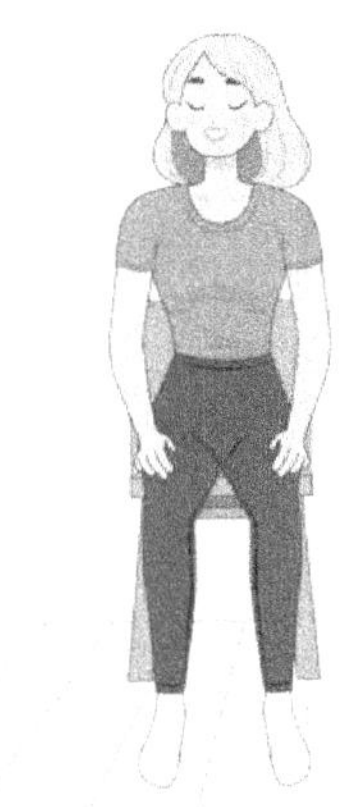

1. Find a comfortable seated position in a quiet space. Close your eyes and take a few deep breaths to settle in.

2. Begin to focus on your breath, noticing the natural rhythm of your inhalations and exhalations.

- You may follow a guided meditation or observe your breath for the duration.

Repetition: Continue this practice for 5-7 minutes, allowing your mind to release any thoughts that arise gently

Caution:

- Ensure you're in a comfortable position to avoid unnecessary strain during the practice.
- Maintain a gentle focus, avoiding over-concentration.

After Exercises: As in previous days.

Week 4: Deepening Practice and Mindfulness

Entering Week 4 of the 28-Day Chair Yoga Challenge, "Deepening Practice and Mindfulness," allows us to take stock of our progress. Week 3 focused on developing strength, flexibility, and coordination; this final week highlights incorporating mindfulness into our practice. Not only do we want to keep getting better physically, but we also want to develop a stronger sense of mental and emotional health. This week is critical in developing a long-term yoga practice because it integrates all the knowledge we've gained for comprehensive training.

The weekly schedule for Week 4 is as follows:

Day	Routine	Goal	Time Spent	Notes
Day 22	Strength-focused Chair Yoga Poses	Build core and upper body strength		
Day 23	Enhancing Flexibility with Deeper Stretches	Improve overall flexibility		
Day 24	Integration of Strength and Flexibility Poses	Balance strength and flexibility		
Day 25	Seated and Standing Poses Combination	Enhance coordination and strength		
Day 26	Focused Breathing with Movement	Synchronize breath with movements		
Day 27	Advanced Seated Twists and Side Bends	Deepen spinal stretches		
Day 28	Review of Week's Poses and Techniques	Consolidate learning from the week		

Day 22: Strength-focused Chair Yoga Poses

Goal: Build core and upper body strength

Before Exercises: 3-5 minutes of Seated Mindful Foundation and breathing exercises, followed by warm-up movements.

DAY 22

EXERCISE	SETS
☐ Chair Dips	x10
☐ Bicycle	x15/side
☐ Side Plank	30sec/side

1) Chair Dips:

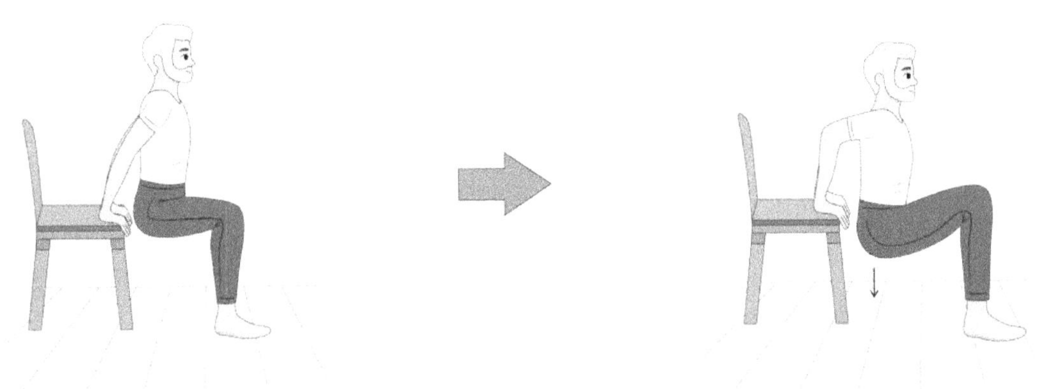

1. Begin by sitting on the edge of a stable chair, placing your hands next to your hips, fingers pointing towards the ground. Your starting position is this seated posture.

● Make sure the chair is secure and won't slide or tip.

2. Slide your hips off the chair and lower your body towards the floor, bending your elbows to a 90-degree angle. Keep your back close to the chair.

3. Push through your palms to straighten your arms, lifting your body back up to the starting position. Focus on engaging your triceps during this movement.

Repetition: Complete a set of ten dips.

Caution:
● Avoid locking your elbows at the movement's top to keep tension on the triceps.
● Control your descent to prevent strain on your shoulder joints.

2) Seated Bicycle Crunches:

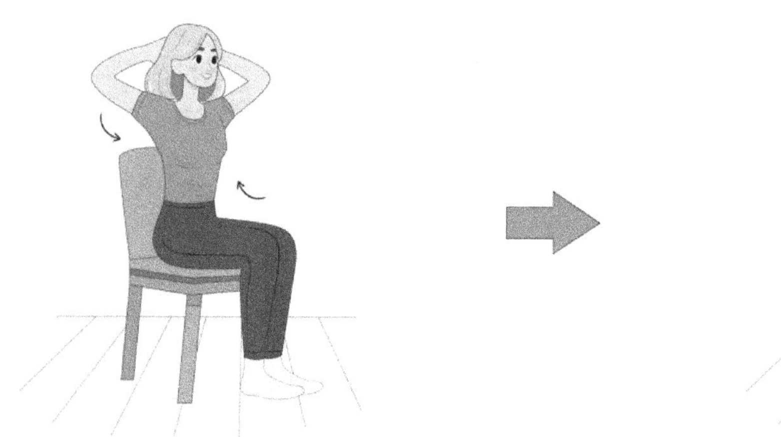

1. Sit back in the chair with a slight recline, placing your hands lightly behind your head without interlocking your fingers. Engage your core to stabilize your upper body.

2. Lift your right knee towards your chest while twisting your torso so your left elbow moves towards the right knee. Extend the opposite leg out.

● Alternate sides smoothly, bringing the opposite elbow towards the lifted knee, mimicking a pedaling motion.

Repetition: Perform 15 repetitions on each side.

Caution:

● Ensure you're not pulling on your neck. Your core should control the movement.

● Keep the movements smooth to avoid jerky motions, which can cause back strain.

3) Chair-Supported Side Plank:

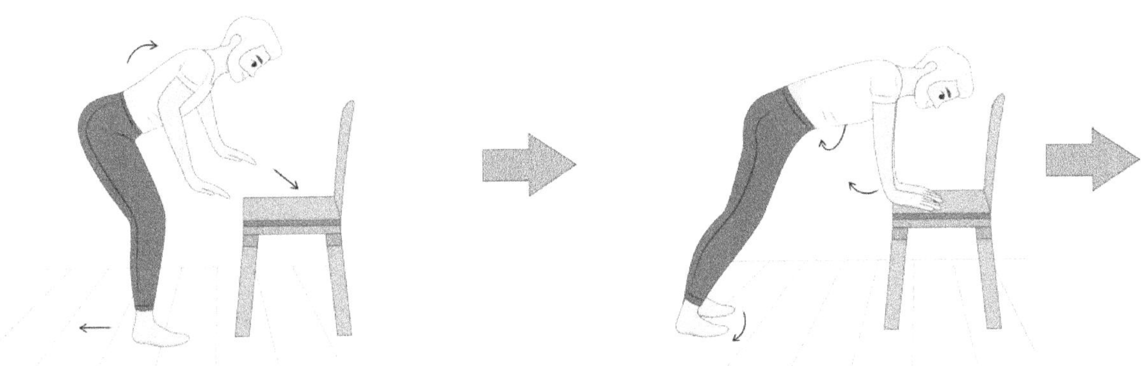

1. Sit beside a chair, placing your hands on its seat for stability. Ensure your feet are side by side or in front of the other to maintain balance.

- Check that the chair is secure and will not slide or tilt.

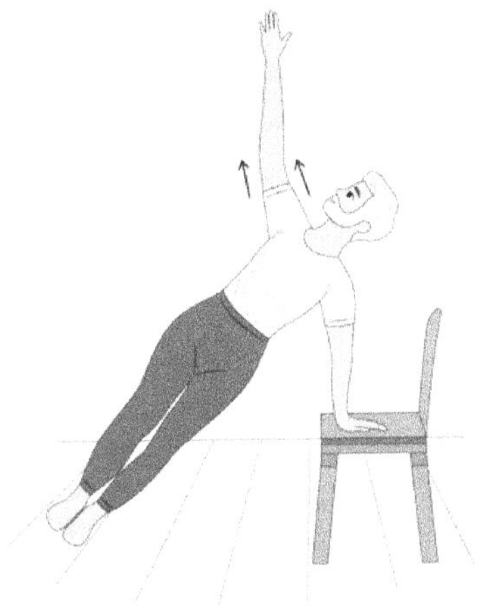

2. Push into your supporting hand to lift your hips, creating a straight line from your head to your feet, forming a "T" shape with your body.

- Engage your core and elevate your hips to form a straight line.

3. Extend your free arm towards the ceiling, keeping your gaze forward or looking at your hand.

- Ensure your neck remains neutral to avoid strain.

4. Hold this position for 30 seconds, focusing on stability and strength in your side body.

- Breathe profoundly and steadily to maintain balance and focus.

Repetition: Maintain the pose for 30 seconds on each side.

Caution:
- Ensure the chair is stable and won't move during the exercise.
- Keep your body straight; avoid letting your hips sag.

Day 23: Enhancing Flexibility with Deeper Stretches

Goal: Improve overall flexibility

Before Exercises: As in previous days.

DAY 23

EXERCISE	SETS
☐ Forward Bend	hold 30sec
☐ Spine Lengthen	hold 30sec
☐ Leg Cradle	15sec/side

1) Seated Forward Bend with Extension:

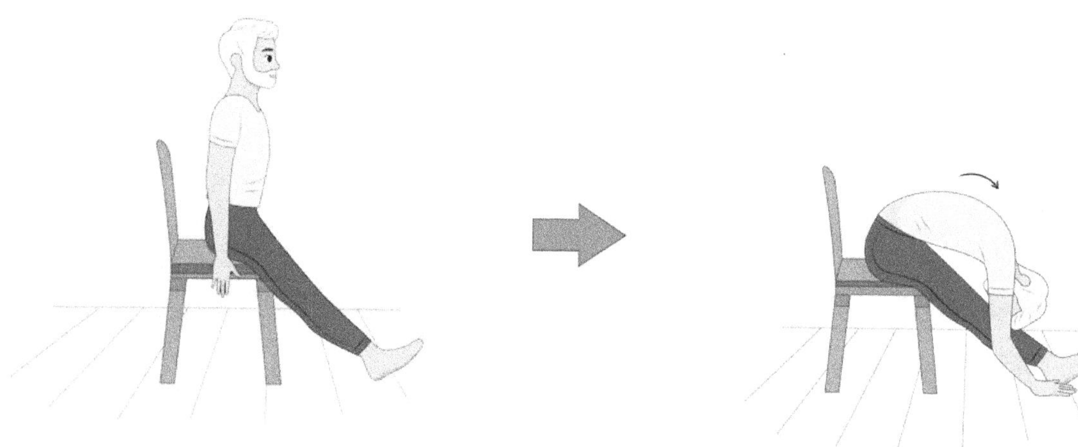

1. Sit with your legs extended straight in front of you. Inhale deeply to prepare.

- Ensure your back is straight and your shoulders are relaxed.

2. Exhale and hinge forward from your hips, reaching toward your toes with your hands.

- Aim to keep your back as straight as possible to maximize the stretch in your hamstrings.

Repetition: Hold for 30 seconds.

Caution: Do not round your back; keep the movement focused on hinging from the hips.

2) Seated Spine Lengthening:

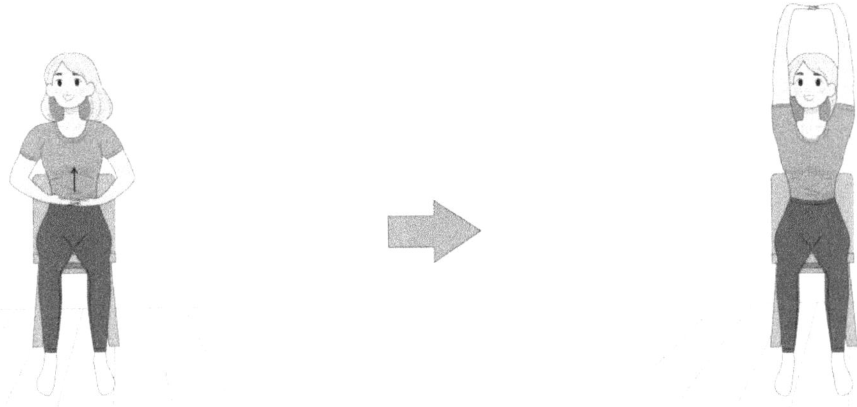

1. Sit tall on the edge of your chair; interlace your fingers and feet flat on the floor.

2. Stretch your arms overhead on an inhale, palms facing up.

● Gently pull your arms back to align with your ears, if possible.

3. Lengthen the spine upwards as if pulled by a string from the top of your head.

Repetition: Hold the stretch for 30 seconds.

Caution: Avoid shrugging your shoulders; keep them relaxed and down.

3) Seated Leg Cradle:

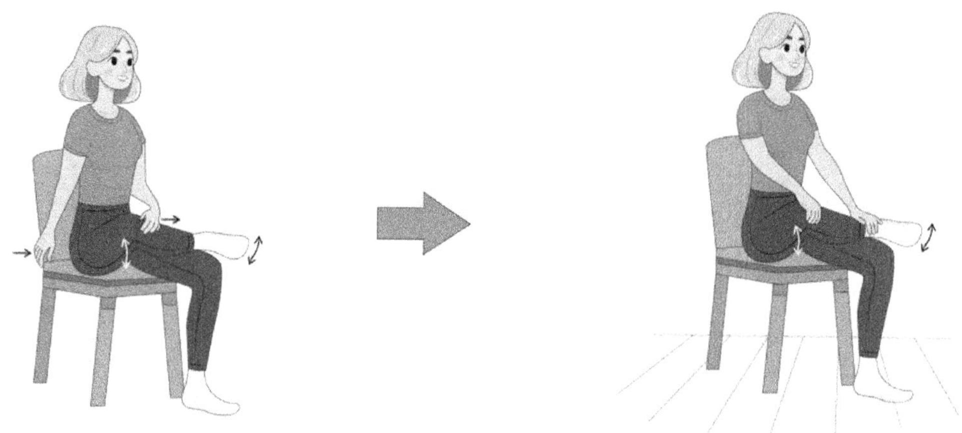

1. Lift your right leg and cradle it with your arms, holding the outer ankle and knee.

● Ensure a gentle grip to avoid putting pressure on the knee.

2. Gently rock your leg side to side to release hip tension.

3. Switch legs and repeat the gentle rocking motion briefly.

Repetition: Alternate legs, spending a few moments on each side.

Caution:

- Maintain an upright posture to prevent slouching.
- Keep the movements soft and controlled to avoid straining the hip joint.

After Exercises: As of Day 22

Day 24: Integration of Strength and Flexibility Poses

Goal: Balance strength and flexibility

Before Exercises: As in previous days.

DAY 24

EXERCISE	SETS
☐ Assisted Lunges	30sec/leg
☐ Warrior Flow	1min/side
☐ Twisting Flow	1min/side

1) Chair-Assisted Lunges:

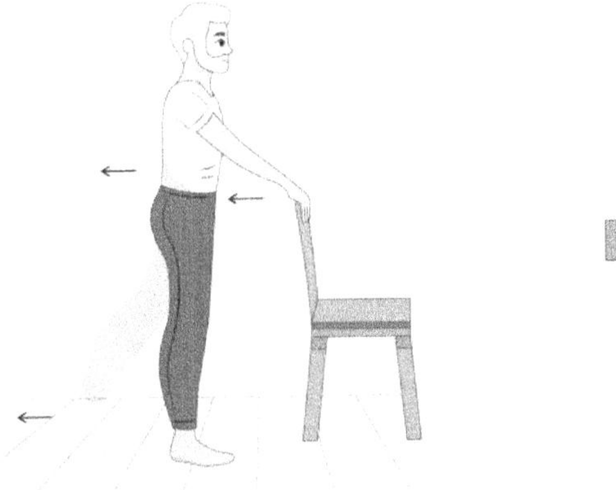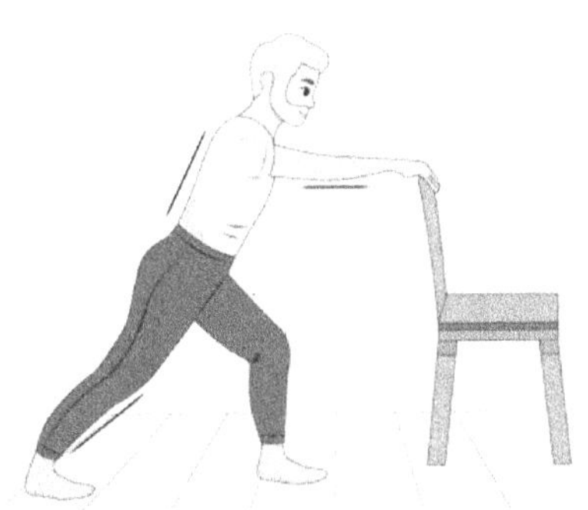

1. Start by standing behind a chair; place your hands on the back chair for support as your feet are hip-width apart.

● Ensure your posture is upright and balanced.

2. Take a giant step back with one foot, entering into a lunge position.

● Your back foot should remain straight and firm on the ground.

3. Bend both knees, lowering into the lunge. Focus on pressing your back toes into the floor to deepen the stretch in your hip.

4. Hold the lunge for 30 seconds and momentarily focus on the stretch in your back leg.

5. Push back up to the starting position and repeat the movement on the other side.

Repetition: Continue alternating sides, holding each lunge comfortably before switching

Caution:

● Maintain balance using the chair to prevent falls.

● Avoid bending the front knee past your toes to protect your knee joint.

2) Seated Warrior Flow:

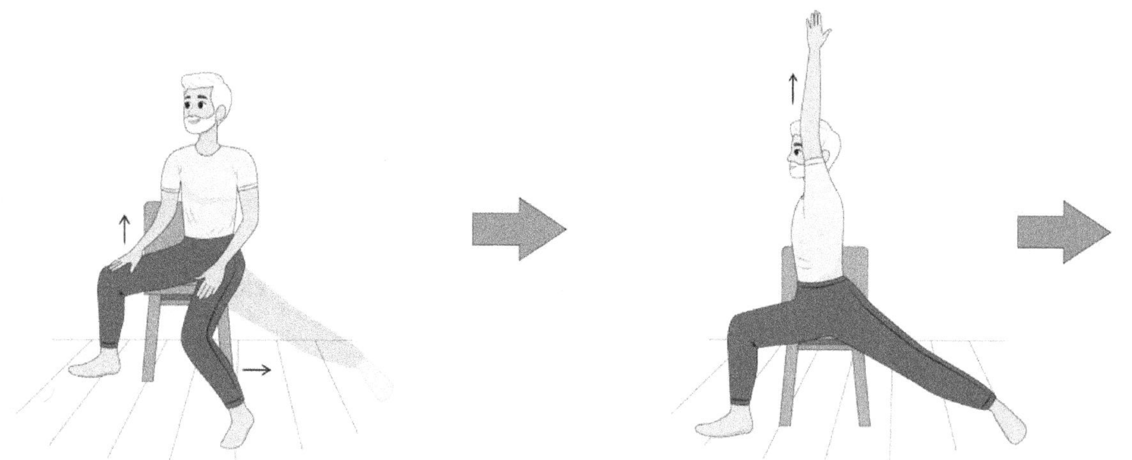

1. Begin seated, slightly forward on the chair, to allow freedom of movement for your legs.

2. Start by positioning one leg ahead with the knee bent and the other leg extended back, mimicking the stance of Warrior I.

3. With a strong base, lift your arms overhead, stretching through your torso. Keep your gaze forward and hips square

● Keep the back leg straight and grounded through the heel.

4. Transition to Warrior II by rotating your torso to face sideways, extending your arms to the sides, parallel to the floor. Ensure your front knee remains bent and directly over the ankle.

● Gaze over your front hand, maintaining a robust and open chest.

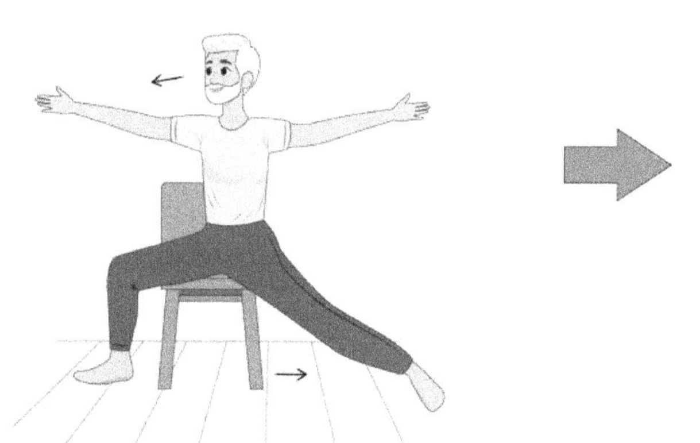

Repetition:

1. **Flow** between these two positions smoothly, coordinating each movement with your breath.

2. Inhale into Warrior I, and exhale into Warrior II.

3. Continue the flow for 1 minute on each side.

Caution:

● Ensure your bent knee does not extend past your toes to protect the knee joint.

● Use the chair for balance, especially when transitioning between poses.

3)Seated Twisting Flow:

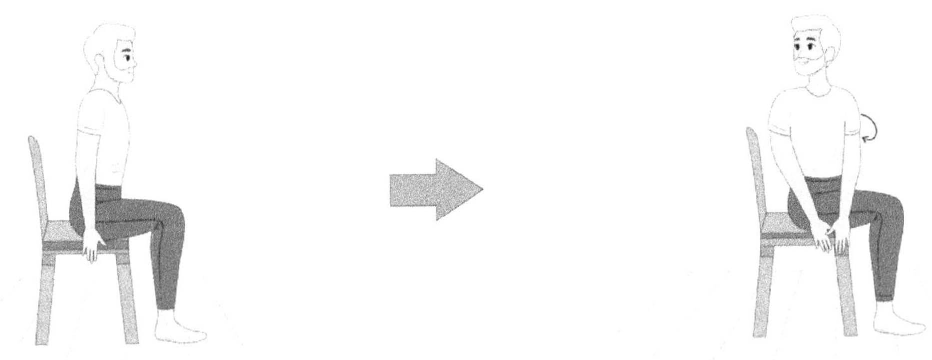

1. Sit is upright in the chair, feet flat on the ground. Place your hands on the sides of the chair for support.

2. Gently twist your torso to the right, using your left hand on the right side of the chair to deepen the twist.

● Keep your spine long and engage your abdominal muscles to support the twist.

3. Return to center on an inhale, and twist to the left side on the next exhale.

● Allow your breath to guide the movement, inhaling back to the center and exhaling into the twist.

Repetition: Hold five deep breaths (30 seconds), then switch sides. Repeat two times

Caution: Twist should be gentle and controlled, originating from the base of the spine

After Exercises: As in previous days

Day 25: Seated and Standing Poses Combination

Goal: Enhance coordination and strength

Before Exercises: As in previous days.

DAY 25

EXERCISE	SETS
☐ Tree Pose	hold 30sec
☐ Squats	x15
☐ Eagle pose	30sec/side

1) Chair-Supported Tree Pose:

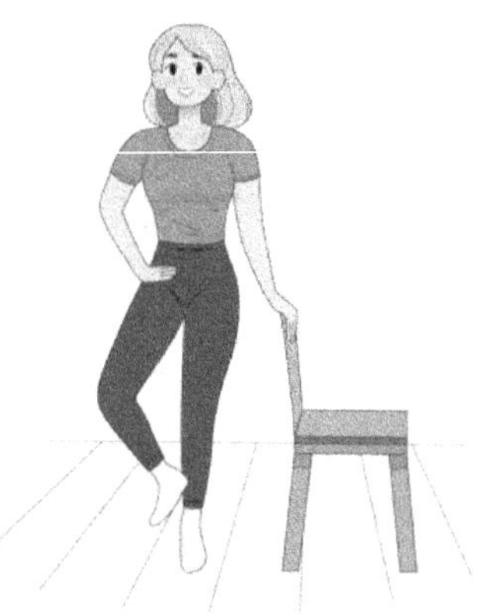
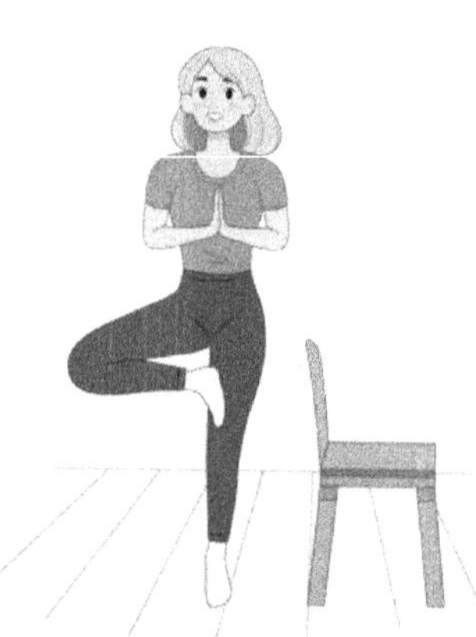

1. Stand beside a chair for balance. Place your weight on your right leg, firmly planting your foot on the ground.

• Place your left foot on your right thigh, avoiding the knee area to protect the joint.

2. With your suitable leg stable, bring your palms together in front of your chest in prayer, maintaining balance and focusing on your breath.

• If balancing is challenging, use the chair for support with one hand.

Repetition: Hold for five breaths on each side

Caution: Use the chair for stability to prevent falls

2) Seated to Standing Squats:

1. Begin seated at the edge of a chair with your feet planted firmly on the ground, hip-width apart

2. Engage your core and leg muscles, pressing through your heels to rise to a standing position.

● Use your arms for balance if needed, extending them forward as you stand.

3. Slowly and with control, lower yourself back into the seated position as if sitting on an imaginary chair behind you with your arms straightened at chest level.

● Control the movement to effectively engage your muscles as you lower yourself back into the seated position.

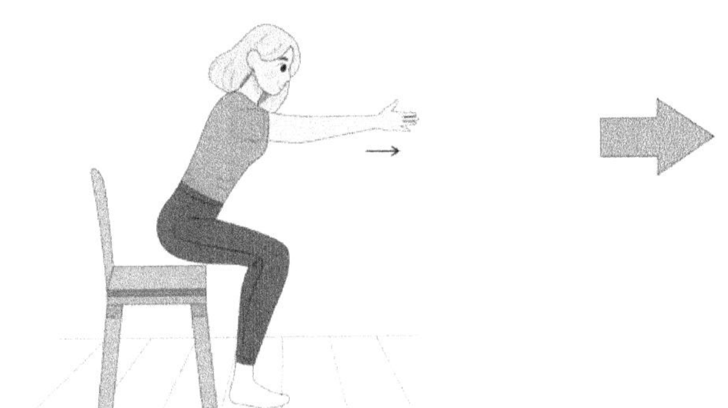

Repetition: Perform 15 repetitions, focusing on strength and control.

Caution:
● Make sure the chair is stable and secure before beginning.
● Focus on engaging your core throughout the exercise to support your back.

3) Seated Eagle Pose:

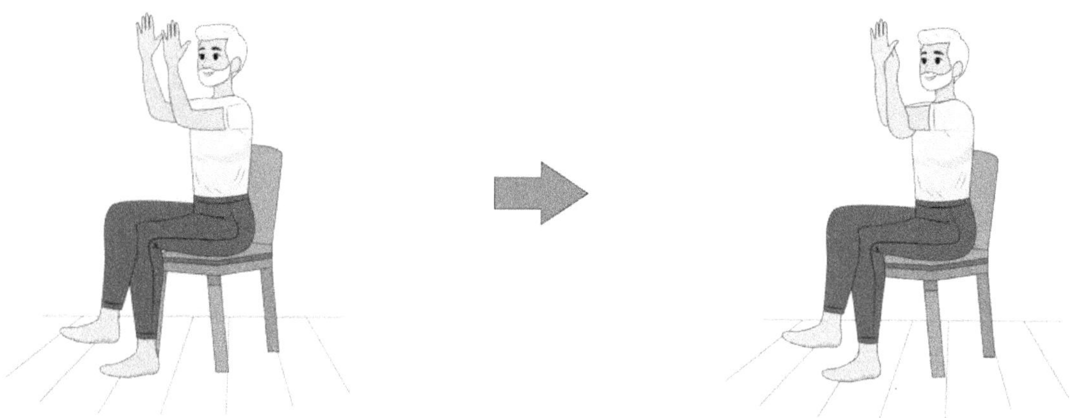

1. Sit upright in the chair, cross your right thigh over your left thigh as much as possible.

2. Bring your left arm underneath your right arm, then bend your elbows to press your palms together or as closely as possible.

● Focus on maintaining balance and alignment in the pose, keeping your spine straight.

3. Hold this position for 30 seconds, breathing deeply and focusing on the stretch in your shoulders and hips.

● Carefully switch sides, repeating the pose with the left thigh over the right and the right arm under the left.

Repetition: Hold for 30 seconds on each side.

Caution:

● Ensure your spine remains straight to avoid slouching.
● Modify the leg and arm positions if you experience any discomfort.

After Exercises: As in previous days

Day 26: Focused Breathing with Movement

Goal: Synchronize breath with movements

Before Exercises: As in previous days.

DAY 26

EXERCISE	SETS
☐ Cat - Cow	2 minutes
☐ Sun Salutation	x3
☐ Guided Breath	3 minutes

1) Seated Cat-Cow with Breath:

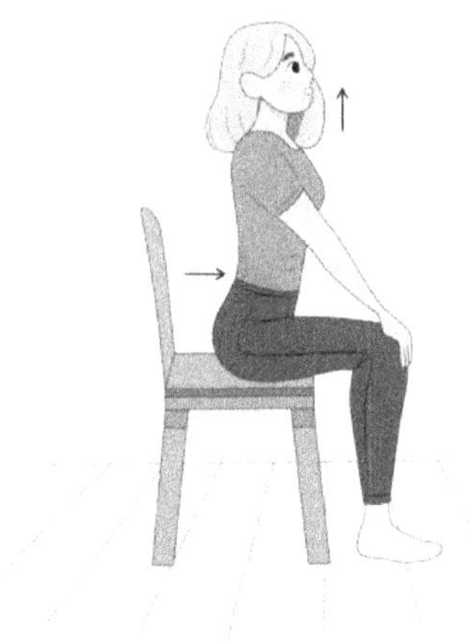

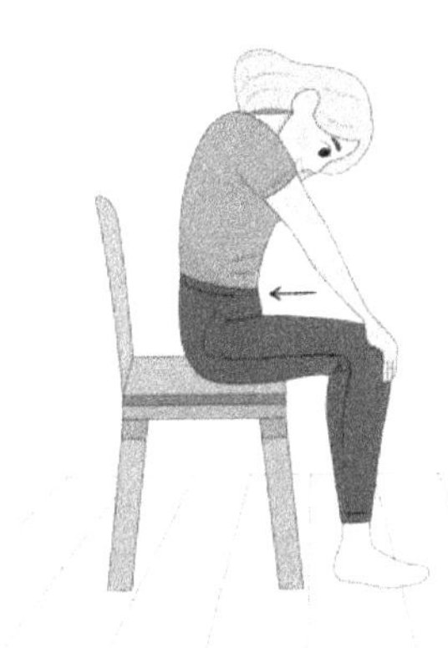

1. Inhale deeply, arching your back and tilting your head and tailbone towards the ceiling (Cow position).

● Ensure a smooth transition into the arch.

2. Exhale fully, rounding your spine, drawing your chin to your chest, and tucking your tailbone under (Cat position).

● Match the rounding of the back with a complete exhalation.

Repetition: Continue for 2 minutes.

Caution: Move gently to avoid any sudden strain on the back.

2) Breath-Focused Chair Sun Salutation:

1. Begin in a seated mountain pose, inhaling deeply.

2. Seated Upward Salute: On your inhale, lift your arms to the sides and above your head, joining your hands if comfortable.

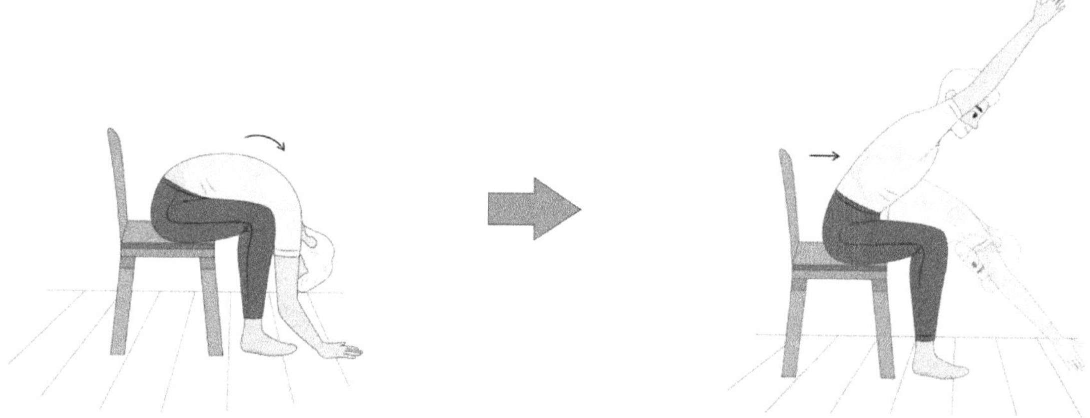

3. Seated Forward Fold: Exhale, hinging at the hips to lean forward, reaching toward your legs. Let your head hang naturally.

● Place your hands wherever they can rest without strain, ensuring comfort.

4. Seated Half Lift: Inhale, lifting your torso halfway up, hands above your head, or on your knees if you feel tension, straightening your back.

5. Return to Seated Forward Fold: exhale and fold again, releasing tension.

Repetition: Repeat for three rounds.

Caution: Ensure each movement is controlled and synchronized with your breath to avoid dizziness.

3) Guided Breathing Exercise:

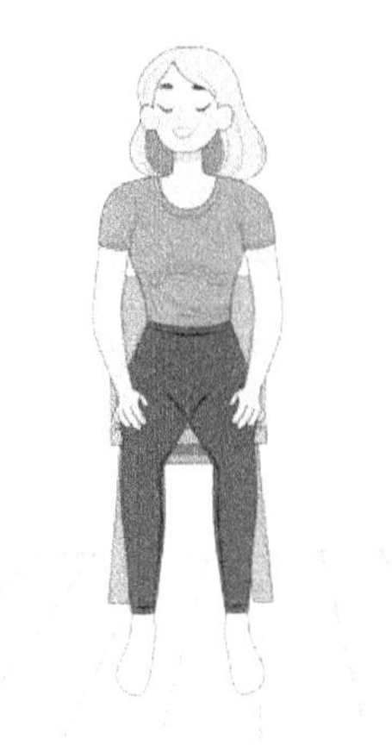

1. Sit comfortably, close your eyes, and begin to notice your natural breath.

2. Inhale deeply for a count of 4, hold your breath for a count of 7.

3. Exhale slowly for a count of 8, fully emptying your lungs.

- Repeat this breathing pattern, focusing on the counts and the sensation of breath moving in and out.

Repetition: Practice for 3 minutes.

Caution: If you feel lightheaded, return to your natural breathing rhythm.

After Exercises: As in previous days

Day 27: Advanced Seated Twists and Side Bends

Goal: Deepen spinal stretches

Before Exercises: As in previous days.

DAY 27

EXERCISE	SETS
☐ Marichyasana	hold 30sec
☐ Side Bend	x15
☐ Seated Twists	30sec/side

1) Seated Marichyasana:

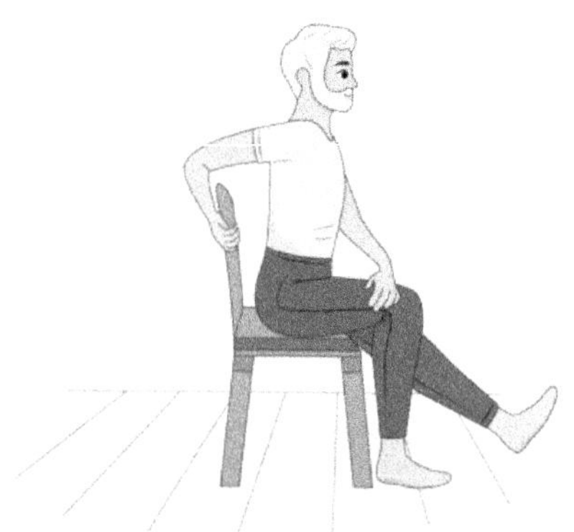 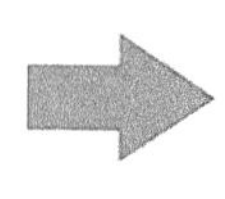 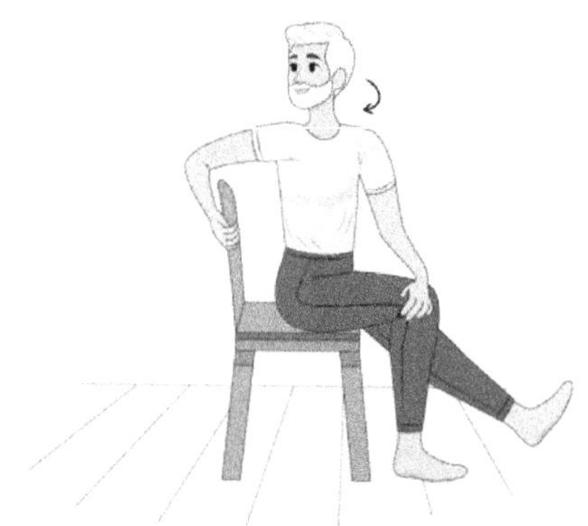

1. Sit with both legs extended in front of you.

2. Bend your right knee, placing the right foot flat on the floor, close to your body.

3. Twist your torso to the right, bringing your left arm over the right knee.

● Use the arm to gently deepen the twist to keep both sit bones on the chair seat.

Repetition: Hold for 30 seconds on each side.

Caution:

● Avoid placing pressure directly on the knee joint during the twist.

● Keep the shoulders relaxed and away from the ears to prevent tension build-up.

2) Seated Extended Side Bend:

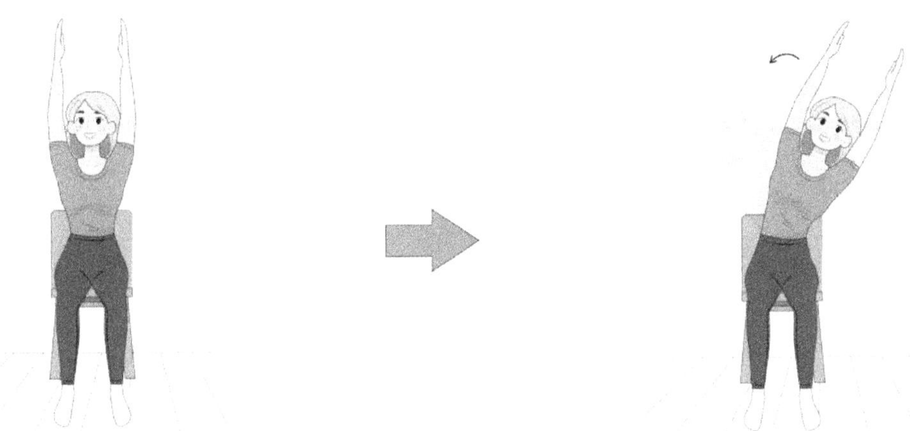

1. Sit upright and extend your left arm overhead, bending to the right side.
• Plant your right hand on the seat or beside your hip for support

2. Push through your right hand to deepen the side bend, stretching the left side of your torso.
• Keep both sit bones firmly on the chair.

Repetition: Hold for 30 seconds on each side.

Caution: Avoid collapsing into the lower side; maintain length on both sides of the waist.

3) Dynamic Seated Twists:

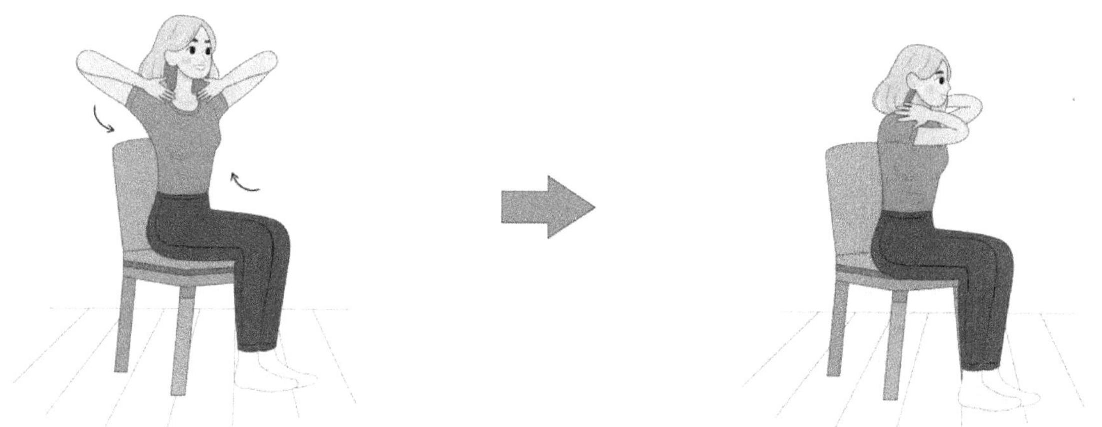

1. Sit flat on the floor and your spine tall. Place your hands lightly on your shoulders.

2. Gently twist your torso to the right, then to the left, creating a fluid, swinging motion.

• Coordinate the movement with your breath, exhaling as you turn to each side.

Repetition: Continue the fluid twists for 2 minutes.

Caution: Ensure movements are controlled and not forced to protect the spine.

After Exercises: As in previous days

Day 28: Review of Week's Poses and Techniques

DAY 28

EXERCISE	SETS
☐ Revisits the most	as in
☐ beneficial poses	previous
☐ from the week	times

Goal: Consolidate learning from the week

Before Exercises: As in previous days.

Routine:
Choose a selection of poses from the week, focusing on those that felt most beneficial. Reflect on the progress made in strength, flexibility, and mindfulness.

After completing the 28-Day Chair Yoga Challenge:

1. Evaluate your experience.

2. Acknowledge how your dedication has enhanced mental clarity, emotional balance, and overall wellness.

3. Consider this not just as the conclusion of an activity but as the beginning of a continuous journey toward well-being.

<u>Chapter 7: Triumphs and Transformation</u>

Congratulations on completing the 28-Day Chair Yoga Challenge! This journey has bolstered your mental, emotional, and physical health and marked the beginning of a transformative path. Embrace the wisdom you've acquired and continue approaching each day with mindfulness and commitment to your well-being.

This experience was far more than a sequence of exercises; it was a profound journey into discovering your inner strength and resilience. Through numerous sessions, you've experienced the benefits of enhanced flexibility, improved balance, and increased awareness—critical elements of chair yoga that enrich everyday life.

Each pose, stretch, and breath has been a step toward a more balanced, healthier lifestyle. You've cultivated awareness and discipline that transcend mere chair exercises, integrating them into your daily routines to navigate life's challenges with a calm mind and a strong body.

Carry forward the valuable lessons and habits you've developed. Let them guide you in times of stress, provide stability amidst uncertainty, and uplift you in moments of joy.

Consider the completion of the 28-Day Challenge not merely as an ending but as the start of a new chapter in your life—a phase for continued exploration, growth, and well-being. This Challenge serves as a motivating beginning to your ongoing journey toward health.

Welcome each day with deep, intentional breaths, embracing gratitude and strength. Stay inspired as your journey continues, promising even more rewarding experiences.

Chapter 8: Everyday Chair Yoga for Seniors

Having completed the rewarding 28-Day Chair Yoga Challenge, you now possess the strength, flexibility, and mindfulness to progress further. Chapter 8 introduces carefully selected chair yoga practices designed for seniors, aimed at maintaining and building upon the gains you've achieved.

The author has crafted these routines to fit seamlessly into your daily life, incorporating a balanced mix of gentle flexibility exercises, strength-building movements, balance-enhancing practices, and comprehensive relaxation techniques. Designed to meet your unique daily needs—whether seeking relaxation, rejuvenation, or overall health and vitality maintenance—these programs allow flexibility to fit your schedule.

Feel free to mix and match different routines for variety or consistently follow those that best meet your physical requirements. Remember, daily mindfulness and consistency are essential. Each day presents a new opportunity to prioritize your well-being, and these routines empower you to do so with joy and ease.

Continue your health and wellness journey with the same dedication and passion you've shown throughout the challenge. Together, let's maintain this path to well-being.

Note: Before performing any of these programs, engaging in warm-up, stretching, and mindful seated foundation exercises is crucial to prepare your body and mind. Each program offers a unique focus, ensuring a comprehensive approach to chair yoga practice tailored to various needs and abilities.

Program 1: Stress Relief & Relaxation (Easy)

Introduction: This program aims to help you unwind and release tension by combining gentle stretches with calming breathing exercises. Duration: 10-15 minutes

Exercises:

Guided Breathing Exercise - Sit comfortably, hands on knees, eyes closed. Inhale deeply through the nose and exhale slowly. (5 minutes) is described in more detail *in Day 26, Exercise 3 on page 119*

Seated Forward Bend - Extend your legs forward and hinge your hips to lean on. Reach towards feet. (3 minutes) in more detail *in Day 3, Exercise 1 on page 54*

Guided Relaxation - Close your eyes, focus on your breath, and follow a guided meditation. (5-7 minutes) *See Day 21, exercise 3 on 103*

Program 2: Flexibility & Mobility (Easy to Moderate)

Introduction: Focus on enhancing your flexibility and joint mobility with these gentle stretches to improve your range of motion. Duration: 10-15 minutes

Exercises:

Seated Spine Lengthening - Sit tall, stretch your arms overhead, and lengthen the spine. (3 minutes) is described in more detail *in Day 23, Exercise 2 on page 109*

Seated Leg Cradle - Gently rock your leg to release hip tension. (2 minutes per leg) *On Day 23, Exercise 3 on page 110*

Seated Twisting Flow - Gently twist your torso to each side, using breath to guide movement. (3-5 minutes) *See day 24, exercise 3 on 113*

Program 3: Upper Body Strength (Moderate)

Introduction: Strengthen your arms, shoulders, and chest with these targeted movements. Duration: 10-15 minutes

Exercises:

Chair Dips - Focus on engaging your triceps. (3 minutes) *On Day 22, Exercise 1 on page 105*

Seated Bicycle Crunches - Engage your core and alternate elbow to knee. (3 minutes) *See Day 22, exercise 2 on page 106*

Chair Supported Side Plank - Engage core and obliques, hold for 30 seconds on each side. (4 minutes) *See Day 22, exercise 3 on page 107*

Program 4: Core Strength & Stability (Moderate)

Introduction: This session aims to engage and strengthen your core, supporting posture and balance. Duration: 10-15 minutes

Exercises:

Seated Marching - Lift knees alternately, focusing on core engagement. (3 minutes) *On Day 16, Exercise 2 on page 88*

Installed Leg Extensions - Extend one leg at a time, focusing on quadriceps engagement. (3 minutes) *See Day 15, exercise 1 on page 84*

Chair Plank - Maintain a straight line from head to heels. (2 minutes) *See Day 8, exercise 1 on page 65*

Program 5: Lower Body Strength (Moderate to Challenging)

Introduction: Build strength in your legs, hips, and glutes with exercises to improve lower body resilience. Duration: 10-15 minutes

Exercises:

Seated to Standing Squats - Focus on strength and control during the movement. (5 minutes) *See Day 25, exercise 2 on page 115*

Chair-Assisted Warrior III - Enhance balance and strengthen the back leg. (5 minutes) *On Day 17, Exercise 2 on page 91*

Program 6: Balance & Coordination (Challenging)

Introduction: Challenge and improve your balance and coordination with poses requiring focus and stability.

Duration: 10-15 minutes

Exercises:

Chair-Supported Tree Pose - Focus on stability and balance; hold for 30 seconds on each side. (3 minutes) *See Day 17, exercise 1 on page 90*

Balanced Walking in Place - Mimic is a marching motion that focuses on lifting knees high and maintaining an upright posture. (5 minutes) *On Day 20, Exercise 3 on page 100*

Chapter 9: Yoga for Specific Conditions

Having mastered the foundational practices outlined in Chapter 8, you now possess techniques to enhance strength, flexibility, and mindfulness. In Chapter 9, "Yoga for Specific Conditions," we delve into the therapeutic potential of chair yoga, expanding upon the exercises introduced in the 28-Day Challenge. Research supports the effectiveness of chair yoga routines in managing and preventing various health conditions, affirming its essential role in a senior's healthy lifestyle[4]. It is important to consult with a healthcare provider before initiating any new exercise program, particularly for those with pre-existing health conditions.

Chair Yoga for Anxiety Reduction

Chair yoga is an invaluable resource for managing anxiety, commonly experienced by seniors. Integrating gentle movements with focused breathing exercises stimulates the body's natural relaxation response, reducing stress hormones and alleviating anxiety-related physical symptoms.

Combating Depression with Chair Yoga

Chair yoga offers a beneficial approach to alleviating depression. Combining physical movement, breathwork, and mindfulness enhances mood, boosts energy levels, and supports overall well-being. The communal aspect of joining a yoga class, even online, provides emotional support and helps combat loneliness.

Emotional Regulation Through Breathing Techniques

Pranayama, the art of yogic breathing, is crucial to mental health. Techniques such as diaphragmatic breathing, alternate nostril breathing, and extended exhalation help calm the mind, reduce stress, and enhance mental clarity.

Managing Common Health Conditions with Chair Yoga:

- **Arthritis:** Increases mobility and reduces joint pain through gentle stretches and strengthening exercises.

- **Heart Disease:** Enhances cardiovascular health by lowering blood pressure, improving circulation, and reducing stress.
- **Diabetes:** Aids in blood sugar control and improves circulation, especially in the lower limbs, by reducing stress and managing weight.
- **Osteoporosis:** Prevents falls and increases bone density through adapted weight-bearing exercises.
- **Chronic Respiratory Diseases:** Targeted breathing exercises improve lung capacity and respiratory health.
- **Alzheimer's and Dementia:** Enhances cognitive function and reduces symptoms of anxiety and depression through mindfulness practices and meditation.
- **Anxiety and Depression:** Utilizes mindful movements and breathing exercises to promote relaxation and tension relief.

Chair yoga is not just an exercise; it's a tool for better health and a pathway to a more fulfilling lifestyle for seniors. Seniors can enhance their mental and physical well-being by integrating chair yoga into daily routines. Always seek medical guidance before starting a new fitness routine, especially if dealing with health issues.

<u>Conclusion</u>

Reflecting on your chair yoga journey, it's clear that this practice transcends mere physical exercises; it embodies a celebration of life's potential at any stage. Chair yoga adapts to your needs, supporting physical and emotional well-being through gentle movements, mindfulness, and meditation.

We've explored how chair yoga enhances mental focus, emotional stability, and physical strength. This journey has been about embracing gentle movement as a transformative power for regaining physical and psychological balance.

Remember, chair yoga is a holistic practice combining physical poses with mindfulness and meditation to enrich your life. Regular engagement with these techniques fosters stress reduction, improved concentration, and respiratory health.

We've emphasized the importance of creating a conducive environment for practice, selecting appropriate equipment, and dressing comfortably to ensure enjoyable and practical sessions. Additionally, adjusting your diet and hydration to support your active lifestyle is crucial for sustaining energy and health during chair yoga.

This journey doesn't end here. The 28-Day Chair Yoga Challenge is just the beginning of continuous personal growth. Embrace this holistic path, weaving mindfulness and physical practice into your everyday life, always attuned to your body's signals and incorporating mindful exercises, proper hydration, and balanced nutrition into your routine.

Carry forward the insights and experiences from this adventure. Chair yoga is more than physical exercise; it's a pathway to enhanced well-being, increased mobility, and deeper self-connection. Embrace each day with open-hearted enthusiasm, celebrating your resilience, strength, and the joy of movement at any age.

Congratulations on completing this transformative journey. May your chair yoga practice and the principles you've learned bring strength, equilibrium, and fulfillment in all aspects of life.

<u>Glossary</u>

1. **Meditation:** A practice of focused attention to increase awareness, reduce stress, and promote calmness and clarity.
2. **Asana:** A term used in yoga to denote various poses or positions. These are crucial for enhancing physical flexibility, balance, and mental tranquility.
3. **Functional Mobility:** The ability to move freely and easily in everyday activities.
4. **Chronic Pain:** Persistent pain that lasts weeks to years, often affecting overall well-being and quality of life.
5. **Pranayama:** Yogic breathing techniques aimed at controlling breath to improve mental, emotional, and physical health.
6. **Holistic Health:** An approach to life that considers multidimensional aspects of wellness, including physical, mental, emotional, and spiritual well-being.

<u>References to Researches</u>

1) *They can also help people with diseases deal with other problems that come with them and improve their quality of life*

Oken BS, Zajdel D, Kishiyama S, Flegal K, Dehen C, Haas M, et al. "Randomized, controlled, six-month trial of yoga in healthy seniors: effects on cognition and quality of life." Altern Ther Health Med. 2006 Jan-Feb;12(1):40-7. This study demonstrates the cognitive and quality of life improvements in seniors practicing yoga.

2) *This is particularly true in senior chair yoga when there are numerous advantages*

McCall T. New York: Bantam Dell, a division of Random House Inc; 2007. Yoga as Medicine.

Desikachar K, Bragdon L, Bossart C. The yoga of healing: Exploring yoga's holistic model for health and well-being. Int J Yoga Ther. 2005;15:17–39

Gatantino ML, Bzdewka TM, Eissler-Rnsso JL, Holbrook ML, Mogck EP, Geigle P, et al. The impact of modified hatha yoga on chronic low back pain: A pilot study. Altern Ther Health Med. 2004;10:56–9

3) *Pranayama includes guided breath awareness, diaphragmatic breathing, and alternate nostril breathing, each offering unique benefits such as improved lung function, stress reduction, and enhanced focus.4*

Joshi KS. *Yogic Pranayama: Breathing for Long Life and Good Health.* India: Orient Paperbacks; 2006

Nivethitha L, Mooventhan A, Manjunath NK. Effects of various *Prāṇāyāma* on cardiovascular and autonomic variables. *Anc Sci Life.* 2016;36:72–7.

4) *Research supports the effectiveness of chair yoga routines in managing and preventing various health conditions, affirming its essential role in a senior's healthy lifestyle*

Yang K. A review of yoga programs for four leading risk factors of chronic diseases. *Evid Based Complement Alternat Med.* 2007;4:487–91